PRACTICE

MADE

PERFECT

Blueprint for a Successful Dental Business

Dr. Michael Dolby DDS, FAGD

*"Elevating the business knowledge of EVERY dentist,
so they can experience owning a profitable, stress-free Practice"*

CONTENTS

4

ACKNOWLEDGMENTS

I would like to sincerely thank the following influential people that have blessed my life:

My amazing wife Katie, for showing me what true love is all about. You gave me the courage and strength to complete this book and believed in me every step of the way. You are my gift from God, and I love you with all my heart.

My awesome children—Connor, Jared, Bella, Max, and Caden. You gave me the gift to love you with all my heart. Each one of you brings a special element to my life that has made me the father that I am today. I love you all soooooooooo much!

My incredible team—especially Cynthia and Sherry, who have been at my side for the past 20 years. Without your dedication, our practice would never have reached and sustained the high level of success we have experienced over the years. You are my family, and I will always be grateful for your friendship, support, and dedication.

My Mom and Dad, my brother, Mark, and my sisters, especially Lisa and Michelle. Thank you for always seeing more in me than I saw in myself.

My wonderful teachers, coaches, and mentors that I have had throughout my life who have provided so many lessons—Paul Pennington, Coach Tony Sutera, Coach Lyle Setencich, Coach Dan Brown, Dr. Jim Makowski, Dr. Tim Dolby, Dr. Dan Fredrickson, Dr. Howard Farran, the amazing UOP Dental School faculty members, Tony Robbins, Steve Moore, and Alan and Sandy Richardson. Thank you for believing in me!

And to all of the wonderful patients I have had the honor to care for, thank you for trusting me with your dental care.

DR. MICHAEL DOLBY

PREFACE

It was 1992, but I remember the event like it was yesterday. I attended my first dental business seminar by Dr. Howard Farran. I was in the middle of my general practice residency program at St. Joseph's Hospital in Denver, Colorado, where I sat in the audience, absolutely mesmerized for the entire program. I took notes as fast as I could write while Dr. Farran listed one amazing strategy after the next. If you have ever had the pleasure of hearing Dr. Farran speak, you know that it's a rapid-fire MBA program and comedy act, all in one.

I initially took his course because I was getting close to the end of my residency and I was trying to discover what my next move would be. What I discovered was my intense passion for the business of dentistry. I loved developing more efficient business systems in the pursuit of creating a stress-free culture while maximizing clinical efficiency and profitability. Unfortunately, what I also discovered at Dr. Farran's seminar was that the majority of dentists in the room was not taking any notes. I couldn't believe it! Here was a guy, hand-delivering exactly how to run a successful, profitable dental practice, and hardly anyone was taking notes. It was then that I made a commitment to learn everything I needed to have an efficient, stress-free, and profitable practice.

In 1994, I bought a practice in Boise, Idaho and began to implement the teachings of Dr. Farran. I worked relentlessly to perfect the business of my new practice. During the day, I cared for patients and focused on the most efficient clinical systems while delivering the highest quality care in the least amount of time. At night, I worked on marketing, branding, and team-building systems to further grow my practice.

In just a few years, I took a practice that was producing $400,000 per year to a practice that was completely insurance-independent and collected over $1,000,000 per year. I accomplished this while working just four clinical days per week, providing greater compensation to my team than did any other office in the area, and keeping my overhead to a very profitable 55 percent.

I have always been drawn towards self-improvement courses, and in 2000

I attended a Tony Robbins seminar. There I discovered that Tony had a company called "Fortune Management." From what I understood, this was a dental management company that combined the best systems in practice management along with the best in Tony's specialty of personal development.

I knew this was something I needed to be involved with, so I made a cold call to a franchisee in Washington. I'll never forget the phone call. An English gentleman answered the phone, and I quickly introduced myself.

"I don't know how I can fit in with Fortune Management, but I want to be a part of it!"

This is how I met Alan and Sandy Richardson, Fortune Management franchise owners. From that day forward, my life outside of clinical dentistry changed. Before I knew it, I was coaching doctors and their teams on how to improve the financial health of their practices, how to build teams that consistently performed at the highest level, and how to realize the goals of the practice while creating a culture that was organized and stress-free.

I was fortunate to be a part-time practice management instructor for PAC Live (Pacific Esthetic Continuum) in San Francisco with Dr. David Hornbrook, Dr. Mike Koczarski, Dr. Ed Lowe, and Dr. Mark Montgomery. In 2005, I took the stage at Discus Dental's Las Vegas Extravaganza where I spoke to more than a thousand people. I feel so blessed to have been presented with these incredible opportunities to teach among the leaders in dentistry. My experience certainly proves that what you focus on, you get.

My passion for the business side of dentistry has continued for more than two decades. Creating and implementing business systems to make the practice as efficient and profitable as possible while providing customer service that is rarely seen in health care is something that gives me unbelievable joy. Unfortunately, there are far too many practices that continue to struggle with the day-to-day management, leadership, and, most importantly, the profitability of their practice.

I set out to create a source where dentists can find solutions to the challenges they face in managing their practices. I documented what I have learned over the past 20 years regarding powerful practice-building strategies and efficient business systems. The result is *Practice Made Perfect—Blueprint for a Successful Dental Business.*

Most of us have heard the advice, *"Find a mentor who has accomplished the kind of success that you want and simply copy that person."* You don't have to reinvent the wheel; just model yourself after your mentor and you will experience similar results. For this reason, I have documented the strategies and systems I have used in my career, so that others can benefit. I have lived and perfected these strategies over the past twenty years, and I know what works and more importantly—what doesn't.

One problem with consultants who have not practiced dentistry is that the strategic plan they create may work on paper, but not in everyday practice. In the real world of dentistry, it is extremely hard work caring for patients, staying on schedule, and managing your team. By following the strategies and tools found in this book, you won't need to reinvent the wheel yourself. My hope is that every dentist will experience a profitable, stress-free dental practice.

I hope you enjoy these stories, tools, and strategies. I look forward to meeting you in person one day and helping your practice become a successful dental business.

Dr. Mike Dolby, *DDS FAGD*

DR. MICHAEL DOLBY

INTRODUCTION

Practice Made Perfect
Blueprint for a Successful Dental Business

DR. MICHAEL DOLBY

WHAT MAKES A DENTAL PRACTICE SUCCESSFUL?

Your purpose explains what you are doing with your life.
Your vision explains how you are living your purpose.
Your goals enable you to realize your vision.
—**Bob Proctor, author and speaker**

Have you ever wondered what differentiates one dental practice from another or why one practice is successful while another struggles when they are in very similar locations?

Early in my career, dentists who separated themselves from the "dental pack" and experienced success were labeled "unethical" or assumed to be "over-diagnosing" and "over-treating." Some were even accused of committing insurance fraud. With that kind of encouragement, who would want to set themselves apart from the others and strive to be ultra successful?

Unfortunately, not much has changed today. Dentists who attempt to break away from the pack are quickly and unjustly criticized.

What we learn in dental school teaches us nothing about how to manage and run a successful dental practice.

I took an unconventional path into dentistry. After high school, I received a scholarship to play football at Boise State University. I wanted to become an architect, but my coaches convinced me that a curriculum like that required too much math and, therefore, was too hard of a major to pursue while playing football. I instead majored in business management, which interested me because of my entrepreneurial spirit and desire to one day own a business.

After graduating from college, I landed a sales position with Beecham Products, a consumer-products company. I was assigned a sales territory, a used Chrysler K-car, and off I went, peddling Aqua-Fresh Toothpaste and

Massengill feminine hygiene products. I hit the ground running, loaded with optimism and eager to prove that I could be a success in business.

As it turns out, I was a little too successful. During my first regional meeting, my district manager pulled me aside and told me that my large sales numbers were making the rest of his team look bad. He then instructed me to only work three days per week and golf the other two days, so that my sales numbers would be in line with the other members of our team … Sounds a lot like the "dental pack" mentality, doesn't it?

This was my first taste of corporate life, and, as you might imagine, I quickly lost interest in the bureaucracy. I began to look for a new career that would allow me to express my creativity and reward me for my hard work. Like many who majored in business, my first thought was about going back to school for an MBA. However, I had no idea what I would do with an MBA when I got it, and hiding out in a classroom for two years seemed like I would just be avoiding making a decision.

I remember sitting at the kitchen table sharing my career frustrations with my stepfather. Out of the blue, he asked, "Why don't you go to dental school?" My uncle was a dentist, but I had never really given dentistry much of a thought. But deep down inside I must have known this profession would allow me to use my creativity while providing me the opportunity to satisfy my interest in owning a business. So without hesitation, I said "yes" and began my quest to become a dentist.

I finally had direction and purpose. Now I just needed to find a way to get accepted into a good dental school.

For some people, school comes easy. You know whom I'm talking about. They rarely study and with minimal effort breeze through classes with amazing grades. This was definitely NOT me.

I have always struggled in school—especially with tests. I seemed to work twice as hard as the rest of my classmates, and my grades were only half as good. My strength was in creativity, which can be hard to assign a letter grade. However, with much determination (and constant pestering of the faculty), I was accepted in the University of the Pacific School of Dentistry in San Francisco. This was my school of choice mainly because of the accelerated curriculum—a four-year program condensed into three calendar years. Once I made the decision to become a dentist, I wanted to take the fast track to accomplish my goal. With a lot—and I mean *a lot*—of hard work, I managed to graduate at the top of my class with high honors. This was an unexpected accomplishment for a former football player with a 2.7 undergraduate GPA.

Dental school taught us the science and clinical skills of dentistry, but very little about how to run and operate a private practice. The only attempt at addressing the business of dentistry was a class that covered vague business principles and what amounted to balancing your checkbook. What was more shocking was the amount of students that struggled in this course. Given the fact that most of the students were science majors, it was no surprise that business topics would be a challenge—just as science was a challenge for me.

Unfortunately, for the majority of these dental students, this was to be the LAST business class they ever took. So it's not surprising that this lack of business savvy follows new doctors into their private practices and throughout their careers.

When I first started helping dentists with the business side of their practices, I found that many doctors had amazing clinical skills but struggled to build a profitable practice. If you have ever attended any of the major dental meetings, such as the American Dental Association's national meeting, you will see the rooms fill up quickly for presentations on the latest crown technique or how to take a superior impression, while the practice management rooms are nearly empty.

It's human nature to be drawn toward what is familiar and to avoid what is foreign. However, the best margins or topnotch cosmetic cases *alone* will NOT make your practice successful. Please don't misunderstand me though. You must have strong clinical skills, or your patients won't stay with your practice, but you must also understand the fundamentals of managing your practice and have specific business systems in place from the moment patients call your office.

So what makes a dental practice successful?

I have found that a practice that implements and emphasizes well-thought-out business systems will perform head and shoulders above the competition. These practices consistently strive to master clinical skills, employ high-performing team members, and use leadership skills to motivate their teams to success.

At Triumph Dental, we have created a simple blueprint for a successful dental practice that is based around three principles: *Foundation, Systems, Leadership™.* When these three principles are implemented, in that order, your practice will reap the same rewards as high-performing practices.

FOUNDATION

This is the framework that your practice will build on. The foundation begins with your identity or brand. This is what you will become known for in your community. Unfortunately, many practices try to be everything to everybody, but that's the quickest way to fail. I will go into this in more detail later, but it's important to identify which areas of your practice you really enjoy and then make that your brand. When we do the things we truly love, somehow it doesn't feel like work, and we remain passionate throughout our career.

Donald Trump claims his success is largely due to surrounding himself with people that are either better than him or masters in a given field. The truth is, that all great businesses assemble team members who perform better as a unit rather than individually. Correctly choosing and training your team is vitally important. The goal is to assemble a team that will consistently support the vision and the mission of your practice while providing superior customer service, all in a stress-free environment.

SYSTEMS

The success of any organization depends on the business systems that have been established. Most dental offices either tend to inherit these systems from previous owners or they have no formal systems at all. This leaves the practice vulnerable to failure. Without systems, patients tend to seek treatment only when they are in discomfort and are less likely to accept your treatment plans or refer their friends and family.

Systems are the tools that your practice will rely on to ensure that every department is operating at the highest level and nothing is missed during the complete patient experience. The implementation of proven business management and personal-development systems will maximize the efficiency and profitability of the practice. It is crucial that every patient experiences the same high-quality care every time they are in your office. Developing systems will allow you and your team to never have an "off day," and you will know where to turn when something in the practice is lacking in performance.

LEADERSHIP

Many dentists say they want someone else to run the day-to-day business responsibilities while they focus on delivering high-quality dentistry. This avoidance of establishing themselves as the leader of the practice is mainly coming from the fear of not understanding how to run a business. The truth is that the owner—the dentist—is the person most at risk financially and so has the most incentive to make sure the practice keeps growing. Your team is looking to you for direction and leadership. This cannot be delegated to a team member or an outside consultant. Every company needs leadership to achieve goals of predictable, stable, and stress-free growth. We all have the ability to lead our teams; we just need to learn how to use the tools that will awaken that hidden leader inside all of us.

Effective leadership will preserve the *Foundation* and *Systems* that you will have worked so hard to implement and will ensure the "little things" are getting done consistently.

What makes a dental practice successful? Follow the principles of success: *Foundation, Systems, Leadership*™. As I break down these three principles and the individual tools to master each one, they may seem small and insignificant by themselves. However, these tools, when implemented together, can mean the difference between success and failure. That is why you will constantly hear me say, *"It takes doing a lot of little things great—CONSISTENTLY!"*™

It is the consistent implementation and management of these tools that will unlock your practice's full potential.

DR. MICHAEL DOLBY

FOUNDATION

Practice Made Perfect
Blueprint for a Successful Dental Business

DR. MICHAEL DOLBY

BUILDING YOUR FOUNDATION

It's not the will to win,
but the will to prepare to win that makes the difference.
—Bear Bryant

All too often, we are so close to our challenges, or the things that hold us back, that we fail to see them and, instead, find ourselves resorting to nothing but excuses.

"There are just too many dentists in my area."

"My patients don't have the financial means."

"The economy is tough on everyone."

Great practices can thrive in tough economic times, even in areas that are saturated with other dentists. These practices look for solutions to their challenges rather than placing blame on things they can't control.

Finding out what your patients want is an excellent way to begin building the foundation of your practice. Every great businessperson must know what their marketplace wants and needs, so they can construct a strategy to satisfy or exceed those wants and needs.

Listed below are the top 10 patient complaints that McGill Advisory gathered back in 2012. I would guess these same patient complaints could be traced back as far as the beginning of dentistry. The easiest way to set yourself apart from the dental pack is to do what others aren't doing. If you know what the people in your marketplace *DON'T* want, then it's easier to give them what they *DO* want.

TOP 10 PATIENT COMPLAINTS

*(According to the McGill Advisory 2012 Newsletter,
Dr. Bill Rossi reported the "Top 10 Online Patient Complaints")*

This report is a sampling of responses from 20 U.S. cities
analyzing over 140 negative reviews.

1. Doctor and staff pushing unnecessary dental services.

2. Poor billing and insurance practices, including hidden or
   deceptive charges.

3. Poor-quality dentistry or incompetent doctor and/or
   staff.

4. Rude and disrespectful front desk staff.

5. Unprofessional staff behavior.

6. Doctor not operating on time; lack of consideration of
   patient time in scheduling.

7. Doctors not compassionate; insensitive to patients.

8. Rushed clinical treatment.

9. Painful treatment.

10. Old, dirty, or uncomfortable office space with out-of-date
    equipment.

Every one of these complaints is based on the defining principle of relationships, or the lack of. When rapport does not exist between you and your patients, there is usually very little value for any of the services you will present to them.

People must feel a connection to you before they will ever trust or buy from you. Just because there is a NEED for treatment doesn't always mean there is a WANT. Dentists often make the mistake of assuming patients will graciously accept their treatment plan simply because there is an obvious need for that treatment. While this may be true when your patient is in pain, once you have solved their immediate problem, value must be created in order for any remaining treatment to be completed. Rapport is the golden rule and must be established first.

BUILDING RAPPORT

Matching & Mirroring

Building rapport is NOT about you. It's not about telling your patients all of your accomplishments in dentistry and why they should feel lucky that you are their dentist. It's about the person in front of you. People buy what they VALUE, and they buy from people they like.

Have you ever met someone you instantly liked or disliked? You immediately either feel connected or distant to this person. Research shows us that people like other people who are just like them. Think about it, your immediate group of friends is very similar to you, right? Similar styles, economic success, the same religion, and similar political opinions.

In the dental profession, we don't have days or weeks to get to know someone. You have about three minutes during an examination to build rapport, so patients will trust you when presenting a treatment plan to them. The best strategy to build instant rapport with someone is called "Matching & Mirroring." It's very easy to do, and the person you are building rapport with never detects a thing. They will just come away with an overwhelming sense that they like and trust you.

This strategy is simple and very subtle. You essentially copy (or match & mirror) the overall presence of your patient. Observe their posture (body language), speech, tonality, breathing, etc. For example, if the person in front of you speaks in a slow, thoughtful manner, then respond in the same manner. If they cross their legs, then you slowly follow suit. If they have a big personality, crank it up a notch to be in sync with them. You get the point. With some practice, you will be able to build rapport instantly with anyone, and they will find themselves drawn to you because *"you are just like them."*

Body Language

When you begin to master the strategy of Matching & Mirroring, focus on the person's body language. We all can say so much about ourselves just by the way we hold our bodies. An athlete will walk into a room in a different manner than a non-athlete. A very feminine girl will hold herself with more poise than a more rugged girl, and so on.

Your goal is not to copy the person exactly, meaning every time they move, you move, because then they will just walk away thinking you're creepy. However, when you recognize a person's body movement, wait about 10 seconds before you mirror their movements. Be conscious of their facial expressions or if they wrinkle their nose, cross their legs, or fold their arms. Use their same hand gestures when it's your turn to talk. You don't have to copy them exactly, but it's important that their subconscious mind ecognizes that you are similar to them.

Tonality & Speed

A person's "tonality" is the sound, pitch, and speed of their voice. Be aware of whether the person you are building rapport with talks loudly or softly. People often talk in one of three ways—through their nose, through their throat, or through their chest. I would never attempt to copy exactly the person's voice or accent. However, I find it most important to follow the tone and speed of their voice. If you are speaking with a loud talker and you talk as if you are in a library, you will have a very difficult time gaining rapport with the person. The same is true if you are speaking to a soft talker and you are speaking much louder and faster than they are. They will recognize, consciously or unconsciously, that you are not congruent, and rapport will be difficult to achieve. They may even view you as annoying and inconsiderate, which obviously will take you further away from being in rapport.

Listen, Repeat, and Approve

The person who is listening during a conversation is truly in the most powerful position. Unfortunately, many people believe just the opposite—that the speaker is in the power position because they are the ones actually talking. Listening isn't just waiting for your turn, so you can get your point across, but engaging what is being said, showing you understand and want to know more. Great listeners learn from the conversations they have with people and are able to connect and build rapport quickly.

It's important to listen for things you have in common with the other person—a place you both lived, a common friend, a similar interest, or maybe a sport you both played. Listening to find that common ground is the key to building rapport.

Then simply repeat and approve what the person said to you. After they speak, summarize what they said with approval words like, *amazing, excellent, great.* A patient may tell you about a trip they just took or a significant event and just respond by briefly recapping what they told you: *"That sounds like an amazing trip"* or *"That part of the country is so beautiful. What part did you like best?"* Asking questions that keep them talking will help you to identify things that you share in common. Most people love to talk about themselves, so make the conversation about them, and you will find rapport can quickly be achieved. My one caveat: Remember, these conversations occur only while your patient is sitting upright, and you are facing them. This strategy is never to be attempted when they are lying on their back with your hands in their mouth—that's just rude!

Assume You Are Already in Rapport

When you are presenting your diagnosis or treatment conference to a patient, assume that you are in rapport with that person. Speak as if you were speaking to a close friend, not hesitant and unsure because you technically don't know them. Subconsciously you will send out signals for the other person to do the same. When you include this with Matching & Mirroring, they will subconsciously feel as if you are both connected in some way. They will see a reflection of themselves through you. When this occurs, you are in instant rapport. The person will not only believe, they will truly feel you have their best interests in mind, which equals trust and trust equals rapport. You can imagine just how much influence you will have on someone once you are in this state, so enrolling your patients into treatment becomes effortless.

Building rapport takes practice and conscious effort but is not difficult to learn. Once you incorporate this system into your practice, you will find that building rapport with patients becomes easy and natural. This strategy works for everyone on your team, regardless of their position.

Everyone on the team should be encouraged to master these techniques to ensure all of your patients feel connected to your practice.

In today's dental environment, we are seeing a patient base that knows they have choices. They can choose where they shop and whom they shop with, including their healthcare providers.

I often hear dentists refer to the "Golden Age of Dentistry" as the best time to practice dentistry. This was back in the early 1970s when dental insurance became available and people for the first time had the Golden Ticket to obtain dental care. The average maximum-allowable insurance benefit for most people during that time was $1,000. When you consider a crown costs just $300 to $400, it was easy to see why a dentist could just hang a sign outside the office and patients would line up around the corner. In fact, people actually had a hard time using all of their dental benefits.

We all know too well that this is not the case today, with the majority of dental plans barely covering basic care. So now, more than any other time in the history of dentistry, we must give potential patients a REASON to choose our practice. We can accomplish this by creating rapport with every patient that walks through the door. Rapport must be strong, so they never have a reason to leave your practice, even when their dental insurance plan tells them they are decreasing their coverage if they stay with your non-participating practice.

You will become more than just their doctor. You will be their trusted friend.

THE POWER OF FOCUS

Always remember: Your focus determines your reality.
—Star Wars Episode I

Have you ever spent months or years saving up enough money to purchase your dream car, and when you finally reached your goal, it seemed like overnight EVERYONE was now driving that exact same car? The fact is, those cars were always there; the only thing that changed was your focus.

What we focus on, we see and often get. It's just that simple. Unfortunately, most people focus on what they DON'T want in their lives, and unfortunately those things show up also. As Dr. Wayne Dyer says, *"Be careful what you focus on because you will eventually get it."*

Most people consider reality to be whatever is in front of them in the moment. How they feel depends on what is happening to them in that moment. Where they are and whom they are with are what determine their emotions. There may be some truth to this; however, we may be in more control of our feelings than we think.

The truth is that what we choose to focus on becomes our reality, no matter what. If you want to feel sad, all you have to do is start thinking of all the messed up things that have happened to you in life, and I guarantee sadness will occur. On the other hand, you also can use the power of focus to make yourself happy. Focus on all the amazing things in your life, and you will find happiness filling your soul.

The Power of Focus, however, is not necessarily instantaneous. When we focus on something we want in our lives, nothing magical happens other than opportunities tend to present themselves, and this will allow you to move towards your goals. You may be unable to recognize these opportunities until your focus is congruent with what you really want to achieve.

I have heard people say, "I really focused on getting a promotion, but it didn't work out." Most likely, they focused on this goal for a few hours, a day, or if they were really ambitious, the weekend, and when they didn't achieve their goal, they gave up. When this happens, the Universe only knows that your focus and energy stopped moving toward your goal.

Therefore, the Universe stopped presenting you with opportunities.

In his book, *Think and Grow Rich*, Napoleon Hill says that one of the most common causes of failure is quitting or losing focus when confronted with temporary defeat. I'm certain every person is guilty of this mistake at one time or another in his or her life, including myself.

Hill tells the story, "Six Feet from Gold," to warn against the lack of focus or quitting too early when a person begins a journey to achieve a goal:

An uncle of R. U. Darby was caught by the "gold fever" in the gold-rush days and went West to DIG AND GROW RICH. He had never heard that more gold has been mined from the brains of men than has ever been taken with a pick and shovel. The going was hard, but his lust for gold was definite.

After weeks of labor, he was rewarded by the discovery of shining ore. However, he needed machinery to bring the ore to the surface. Quietly, he covered up the mine, retraced his footsteps to his home in Williamsburg, Maryland, and told his relatives and a few neighbors of the "strike." They pooled together money for the needed machinery and had it shipped to the mine.

The first car of ore was mined and shipped to a smelter. The returns proved they had one of the richest mines in Colorado! Just a few more cars of that ore would clear the debts. Then would come the big killing in profits.

Down went the drills! Up went the hopes of Darby and his Uncle! Then something happened. The vein of gold ore disappeared! They had come to the end of the rainbow, and the pot of gold was no longer there! They drilled on desperately trying to pick up the vein again but to no avail.

Finally, they decided to QUIT. They sold the machinery to a junk man for a few hundred dollars and took the train back home. Some "junk" men are dumb, but not this one! He called in a mining engineer to look at the mine and do a little calculating. The engineer advised that the project had failed because the owners were not familiar with the "fault lines." His calculations showed that the vein would be found JUST THREE FEET FROM WHERE THE DARBY'S HAD STOPPED DRILLING, and that is exactly where it was found!

The "junk" man took millions of dollars in ore from the mine because he knew enough to seek expert counsel before giving up.

DR. MICHAEL DOLBY

DELAYS ARE NOT DENIALS

Never, never, never quit.
—**Winston Churchill**

Imagine this: You wake up in the morning and think about all the patients you need to see later in the day. Your focus is entirely on those miserable, ungrateful patients, and you just can't get them out of your head.

Because your focus creates your reality, most likely you will create exactly what you feared, and a miserable day is certain. On the flipside, if you wake up and focus on what a wonderful gift your life is and how lucky you are to have the skills to care for your patients, you are certain to have a great day.

Our thoughts create our feelings, and our feelings create our reality. Therefore, wherever our mind (focus) takes us, that reality has a strong possibility to manifest around us. With this understanding comes great power, so we must be cautious on where our thoughts lie because we know this can work *for* us—or *against* us. It's OUR CHOICE.

When we let our attention jump from one thing to another, we will most likely experience a busy, fractured, and probably unproductive day. Have you ever had a time in your life when you have been so focused on a project that you lost all sense of time, barely ate or used the restroom? You probably made great progress and had a rewarding day.

So how do we use this Power of Focus in our everyday lives, especially in our dental practices?

We achieve this through visualization. Whatever we can see in our mind, we can create. For example, let's say you would like to see a $100,000 production month. You can begin first by closing your eyes and relaxing your mind. Take a few deep breaths and picture yourself at the end of the month looking at your production numbers. See yourself holding that production sheet and seeing the number $100,000. Imagine what it's like to achieve this goal. Take in this sensation of success and acknowledge how great it feels.

Now take a step back and reflect on how you arrived at this goal. Watch yourself in your morning team meetings with a full, productive schedule. See yourself while presenting your treatment plans, building instant rapport, and watching as your patients accept all of your recommended treatments. Witness your team offering unprecedented customer service, and watch how your patients are passionate about referring their friends and family.

This is how easy it can be to achieve any goal—when you can see it first in your mind. There are some who say your mind is incapable of seeing something it can't achieve. So if you can see it, that means you can achieve it.

When you repeat this visualization exercise over and over, you will convince your brain that this is not only possible, your brain will actually think you have already reached this level of accomplishment. By doing this simple strategy, you will dramatically increase the speed of achieving any goal. Isn't it true that when you have already achieved a certain goal, that it's so much easier the second time to get back to that level again? I have seen doctors with million-dollar practices sell those practices and start in a completely new location where others have struggled, only to repeat the process of creating a million-dollar plus practice. Why? Because they have done it before and their brains know of nothing else.

Knowing you have this power, can you imagine how quickly you can change the way you feel and make progress towards your goals? Remember, you have all the power inside of you already to choose your destiny, so make the right choice!

All that we are is the result of what we have thought.
—Buddha

VISION & MISSION STATEMENTS

So many of our dreams at first seem impossible,
then they seem improbable, and then, when we summon the will,
they soon become inevitable.
—Christopher Reeves

The Vision & Mission Statements are unfortunately an underutilized, but important, part of building your foundation. Taking the time to think about what you want to accomplish in your practice and career is far too important to put aside. Dentists often rush into their practice focused entirely on the clinical aspects of what they want to accomplish. They are so excited to start preparing crowns and learning to place implants or buying a new Cerec machine that they lose sight of the meaning or legacy of their practice.

At the end of your career, you want to know that what you accomplished mattered and that the direction you chose for your practice had meaning and was not based on random outcomes or trends.

Your Vision & Mission Statements are the words you choose to describe the direction and meaning of your practice. By creating a clear vision for your practice, you will powerfully communicate your intentions and motivate your team to realize that vision.

Vision: Outlines what the organization wants to be or how it wants the world in which it operates to be known for. (An "idealized" view of the world.) It is a long-term view. It can be emotive and is a source of inspiration. For example, a charity working with the poor might have a vision statement that reads, *"A world without poverty."*

Mission: Defines the fundamental purpose of an organization or an enterprise, describing why it exists and what it does to achieve its vision. For example, the charity above might have a mission statement, such as *"Providing jobs for the homeless and unemployed."*

"MISSION STATEMENTS" – VS. – "VISION STATEMENTS"

Your Vision Statement defines your purpose from a broader view. It is the practice's values rather than bottom-line measures. (Values are guiding beliefs about how things should be.) A Vision Statement is something you want to become or achieve. It is your image of an ideal future.

The Vision Statement communicates both the purpose and values of your practice. For your team members, it provides direction regarding how they are expected to conduct themselves and inspires them to give their best. This becomes the foundation for the culture of your practice. This will also direct your patients' understanding as to why they chose to have you care for their dental needs. A Vision Statement defines who you are and what you are about.

A Mission Statement defines the purpose of your practice. Its main function is to define why your practice exists and how this supports your vision. You can think of a Mission Statement as your action plan to realizing your vision.

CREATING YOUR VISION STATEMENT

First identify how you want others to view or talk about your practice. How do you want to be known in your community? Use emotional words that have meaning for you and your team.

Next you will identify what your team and your patients value most about your practice. Use words describing your Vision that are inspiring enough to energize and motivate your team to support and live by this vision.

Take time with your team to brainstorm the words that describe this Vision for the practice. Write it down, post it in the break room, and commit it to memory.

1. Identify how you want others to perceive your practice. How do you want to be known in your community?

2. Identify what you and your patients will value most about your practice.

3. Use words in your Vision Statement that are inspiring enough to energize and motivate your team.

Here are some examples of Vision Statements:

Nike
Vision Statement:

1960s: *Crush Adidas*
Current: *Be the number one athletic company in the world.*

Pfizer
Vision Statement:

At Pfizer, we're inspired by a single goal: your health. That's why we're dedicated to developing new, safe medicines to prevent and treat the world's most serious diseases. And why we are making them available to the people who need them most. We believe that from progress comes hope and the promise of a healthier world

Boeing
Vision Statement:

1950s: *Become the dominant player in commercial aircraft and bring the world into the jet age.*
Current: *People working together as one global enterprise for aerospace leadership.*

Triumph Dental
Vision Statement:

Elevating the business knowledge of EVERY dentist, so they can experience owning a profitable, stress-free practice.

CREATING YOUR MISSION STATEMENT

Write your Mission Statement with the goal of being an action, not a sentiment, and one that is quantifiable, not nebulous. If you're trying to change people's lives, how are you going to do that? Whose lives are you going to change?

Create your Mission Statement by first identifying the "purpose" of your practice. Your purpose makes your practice stand out from competitors. It is the reason that new patients will seek you out. Use strong emotional words that have meaning for you and your team.

Next, identify the key measures of your success. Make sure you choose the most important measures and not too many of them.

Combine your purpose and success measures into a measurable goal. Write and rewrite until your Mission Statement reflects the difference that you want to make, and post it in the break room and commit it to memory.

1. To create your Mission Statement, identify the purpose of your practice.

2. Your purpose is what will make your practice stand out from competitors. It is the reason that new patients will seek you out.

3. Identify the key measures of your success. Choose the most important measures and not too many of them.

4. Combine your purpose and success measures into a tangible and measurable goal.

5. Write and rewrite until it reflects in words the difference that you want to make.

Here are some examples of Mission Statements:

Nike
Mission Statement:

To bring inspiration and innovation to every athlete in the world.
"If you have a body, you are an athlete."

Pfizer
Mission Statement:

We will become the world's most valued company to patients, customers, colleagues, investors, business partners, and the communities where we work and live.

Boeing
Mission Statement:

"Run healthy core businesses. Leverage strengths into new products and services. Open new frontiers. People working together as a global enterprise for aerospace leadership."

Triumph Dental
Mission Statement:

Providing select dentists a clear path to ownership, teaching them everything they need to know to operate and manage a profitable, stress-free dental practice.

Writing your Vision & Mission Statements can be relatively easy while implementing these into your practice can often present a challenge. Your Vision & Mission Statements should be used as a leadership tool to promote change in your practice and move you toward your goals while aligning your team's performance to match your Vision & Mission. Reviewing this consistently is the key to creating a culture that supports these goals.

JOB DESCRIPTIONS

My philosophy is that not only are you responsible for your life, but doing the best at this moment puts you in the best place for the next moment.
—**Oprah Winfrey**

Why are job descriptions so important? A dental assistant or hygienist obviously knows what to do, right?

Right!

I get that response from some doctors, and unfortunately their practices are usually suffering. The reason is that the team members are not sure of their exact responsibilities. Creating a detailed job description for every team member eliminates any assumption of who does what and when. This is crucial for any team to reach its maximum potential.

All job descriptions must be included in your practice's employee handbook, and using these job descriptions during the hiring process for new team members is essential. Candidates need to understand the job duties and know exactly what is expected of them.

Job descriptions should also be updated for each team member during the annual review. As your practice changes and grows, so do the responsibilities of your team members. It's important to keep these job descriptions up-to-date.

A creative and, more importantly, effective way to begin writing job descriptions is to get your team involved in the process. Ask them to write down their own job descriptions from their perspectives first. You may be surprised at the amount of misunderstanding about the job duties you think they should be responsible for and the ones they think they should be doing. You also might find areas of accountability that are either duplicated or not addressed at all. Delegating these responsibilities to the appropriate team members will make the practice more efficient and essentially more profitable.

Once you have your team members' input, start developing each job description with the purpose of the team member's position in the practice along with a list of the duties that are associated with that position. Be specific, so no detail is ever assumed. Lastly, describe the special skills, qualifications, or certifications that are required for the position.

Create a master job description for each department and have team members sign their respective job descriptions, so they take full responsibility to uphold those duties.

EXAMPLE JOB DESCRIPTIONS

Description: Dental Assistant

Dental Assistant Purpose: Supports dental-care delivery by preparing treatment room, patient, instruments, and materials; passing instruments and materials; performing procedures in compliance with the Dental Practice Act.

Dental Assistant Job Duties:

- Lead dental assistant is responsible for all ordering of dental supplies and documenting these orders. Not to exceed 5% of total net collections.

- Awareness and application of infection control.

- Makes all types of temporary restorations.

- Completes chart documentation of treatment with correct fees and tooth numbers.

- Responsible for encouraging patients to complete outstanding treatment.

- Education and delivery of bleach trays.

- Informs all patients of treatment being completed that day along with treatment needed.

- Reviews all post-op instructions with patients along with providing patients with the proper post-op instruction sheets.

- In-depth knowledge of tooth morphology and numbering system.

- General knowledge of pharmacology and prescription writing.

- Administration and knowledge of N2O2.

- Knowledge of dental anesthetics and various dental materials.

- Takes accurate alginate and final impressions, along with bite registrations.

- Placement of dental sealants.

- Denture and removable partial-denture adjustments.

- Makes bleach trays, sports mouth guards, and night splints.

- Creates patient rapport, and puts patients at ease before treatment.

- Deals with special needs patients in a positive, caring, and professional manner.

- Maintains CPR training.

- General knowledge of all restorative techniques and instruments.

- Maintenance and upkeep of all equipment.

- Lab Duties: pouring, trimming, labeling, and storage of study models.

- Tracks and logs all lab cases.

- Greets and dismisses patients in a courteous and professional manner.

- Patient education.

- Takes x-rays/ bitewing, PA, Panorex, mounting x-rays correctly.

- Educates patients on the advances in cosmetic dentistry.

- Consistently provides OUTSTANDING customer service while asking for referrals.

Skills/Qualifications:

Demonstrates complete understanding of dental terminology; familiar with current dental technology; trained with current infection-control protocol; provides outstanding customer service; excellent listening skills; works well with other team members; shows ability to build rapport with patients; promotes the practice in the community.

BECOMING A GREAT TEAM MEMBER

When you judge another, you do not define them, you define yourself.
—**Wayne Dyer, psychotherapist**

Being part of a TEAM is the greatest feeling in the world. A group of individuals working together for a common goal is more powerful than any talented individual working alone. It's an awesome feeling when your teammates are depending on your performance to help achieve the team's goal. The feelings of significance and love run through your entire body.

When we think of teams, our minds often relate to sports teams, especially when it comes to the underdog. That's the team with the so-called weaker, less-experienced individuals that somehow manage to defeat the favored all-stars.

So how does a group of average athletes defeat a group of more talented ones? A team succeeds when all of its members share the same goal. They all focus on one outcome, no matter what hurdles they face. That is why you see teams that may be behind on the scoreboard, but the team's overwhelming confidence that they will be victorious leads to exactly that outcome: victory. A group of individuals whose concentrated focus on a common goal will most likely defeat a group of individuals with no goal at all.

In our dental office we have the same opportunity to come together as a team and experience the success of being more effective together than individually.

WHAT MAKES A GREAT TEAM?

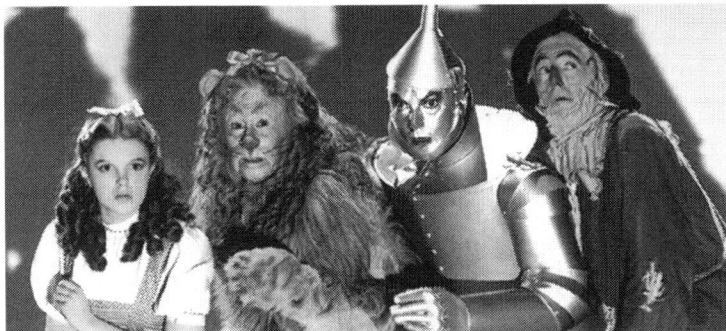

Great people make a great team, right? That's true, but it depends on how you define "great."

Unfortunately, many dental practice owners get it wrong. They assume a great team member is someone who has a vast amount of experience with your particular practice management software or a dental assistant who can make amazing temporaries. These people may be great individually at those certain tasks, but the practice may still suffer if these individuals are unable to work as a team towards a common goal.

The film, *The Wizard of Oz*, in my opinion, is the best team-building parable in movie history.

A Kansas farm girl, Dorothy, is sucked into a tornado and dropped into the magical Land of Oz. Her "landing" in Oz accidentally kills the Wicked Witch of the East, which creates a powerful enemy—the Wicked Witch of the West. On her quest to return home to Kansas, Dorothy travels down the Yellow Brick Road to seek help from the great and powerful Oz. Along the way, she meets the Scarecrow who wants a BRAIN, the Tin Man who is in search of a HEART, and the Lion who desires COURAGE.

They share a common goal of reaching the powerful Oz, so he may grant them their wishes. This oddball team overcomes incredible odds and kills the Wicked Witch of the West only to discover that the great and powerful Oz is not so great and powerful after all. However, Dorothy and her friends discover a truth that is more powerful than any magic: Everything they desired—brains, heart, courage, and the ability to return home—had been right inside of them all along. They had to look no further than within themselves.

In the end, the power of a team was greater than any individual—including the Wicked Witch of the West.

"THE WIZARD OF OZ" LESSONS FOR TEAM MEMBERS:

- Assemble a diverse team.
- Work toward a clear goal.
- Encourage the greatness of your team's natural talent.
- Keep moving forward, especially when things get tough.
- Be conscious of the resources that are already in front of you.

TOP TEN QUALITIES OF A GREAT TEAM MEMBER

(1) Friendly
(2) Reliable
(3) Communication Skills
(4) Customer Service
(5) Flexible
(6) Problem-Solver
(7) Respectful
(8) Proactive
(9) Strive to be an Expert
(10) Laugh, Live, and Celebrate

FRIENDLY

This is the first and most important quality to look for in any team member. You cannot teach someone to be friendly, and this certainly should not be overlooked. Do not make the mistake of being swayed by a person's clinical or front office skills and think that you will be able to teach them to be friendly and make patients feel welcome in your practice. This will never happen, at least not consistently. I will always take a personable, outgoing, friendly person over a technically skilled person. I can teach you the technical stuff, but I can't teach you to be nice.

How can you tell if someone is friendly? Watch how they interact with other people. Observe how they address you when meeting for the first time. Did they greet you with a handshake and a smile while making eye contact, or were they nervous, shy, and unsure?

You need every member of your team to be outgoing and happy, so that your patients feel relaxed when they are in your office. The practice of dentistry comes with enough negative connotations, and we certainly don't need anymore, especially coming from your own team members.

RELIABLE

Great team members are employees you can count on. They show up to work on time and have prepared themselves for the day. They say what they mean and mean what they say. They are RELIABLE. There is nothing more challenging than a non-reliable team member.

How can you tell if someone is reliable? You can ask, "How many continual days of attendance at work would you consider satisfactory? How many days of work did you miss last year?"

They should answer, without hesitation, that all team members should make it to work on time every day unless there is an emergency in which they would notify the appropriate person with as much notice as possible. Great team members want to be punctual and consider attendance an important part of their job description.

COMMUNICATION

Effective communication is an important quality when running a busy dental practice. Communication among team members and with patients is crucial to the success of your practice. Every team member has a responsibility to master effective communication in order to create VALUE for the services you are offering. Communication leads to rapport with your patients, who are evaluating every aspect of your team—especially how members communicate with each other.

People communicate with each other for three primary reasons: (1) It makes us feel good. (2) It is a cry for help. (3) It is an attempt to see a "new result."

Effective communication in your office should accomplish the following: (1) make your patients feel good; (2) make your team feel good; and (3) create value for your patients.

Most people think that words are the most important part of communication. We worry so much about choosing just the right words to say to our patients, which can sometime cause us to memorize lines that don't end up conveying the message we are actually trying to communicate.

Did you know that words only account for approximately 7% of the effectiveness in our communication? While tonality accounts for an impressive 38% of our communication effectiveness, and physiology (our body language) accounts for a whopping 55%. This is clear evidence that it's more important HOW you say something, rather than the actual words you use.

Think about someone who is very excited about what they are saying to you. Their body language and tone of voice speak volumes. Don't you find yourself more engaged and interested in what they have to say? Your answer is probably "yes."

Communication is both verbal *(words - tonality)* and nonverbal *(physiology - environment.)*

Verbal communication is when our words are accompanied by our tonality, or the speed and pitch of our voice. This is really important when we are speaking to a patient over the phone. In the obvious absence of our nonverbal physiology, we must master not only our words but also the tone in which we use them. Strive to be congruent with the tone of the person you are speaking with. As I said before, the quickest way to be in rapport with someone is to match and mirror their behavior, which includes the tonality in their voice. When speaking to a person who uses a soft tone of voice, the last thing you want to do is speak in a loud tone. This will create disconnect with the person you are speaking with and make it extremely difficult to build rapport or a sense of bond.

Nonverbal communication is the expression of words through body movements, and, as stated before, this is the most powerful form of communication.

When we add excitement to our communication, it often raises the level of curiosity with the other person and engages them in the conversation. When you are presenting a treatment plan to a patient and you include excitement and optimism, I guarantee your case acceptance ratio will improve.

People are attracted to people who are excited about their lives and their work. However, you must base your level of excitement on the nonverbal physiology of the other person. Even still, adding a little excitement to your conversation through gestures and body movement can often raise the level of excitement of a passive or soft-spoken person.

Nonverbal communication can be positive as described above or negative. If a patient arrives at your office on time for their appointment and you unintentionally make them wait because you are off schedule, it can only communicate a negative message that your time is more valuable than theirs. Or when was the last time you updated the furniture, wall colors, and other decor in your office? Does your office look old and run-down or does it represent the quality and professional environment you are striving to create? Better yet, what is the condition of your smile or your team members' smiles? If they have not been restored to the quality that you promote to current patients in your practice, that can be viewed as a negative message.

So how can you tell if a prospective team member is a good communicator?

Ask them, *"What steps do you take to create rapport with others?"*

The answer should be that they see things from another person's perspective and are willing to discover things they have in common. Can this person empathize with patients? Empathy is an essential component to building rapport.

Ask the prospective team member to give you an example of the last time they had to present a complex treatment plan in simple terms. You want to hear them describe how they broke down complex information in order to help patients reach a complete understanding of the treatment proposed.

A good communicator is someone who is curious and responsible enough to care that his or her message is being heard and understood, and can work with many different personalities. They are flexible and do not get flustered when the other person is having a difficult time understanding what they are saying.

CUSTOMER SERVICE

Customer service is more than a nice waiting room with a coffee bar and the most current magazines. And it's certainly more than having the most up-to-date, high-tech dental equipment to show off. Outstanding customer service is more than what you DO for your patients, as it is defined by the CULTURE that is created within your practice.

Have you ever walked into a business and immediately felt unsure or just not comfortable? How about a walking into a new restaurant and before you actually spoke to anyone, you immediately felt at home and welcome? This is the culture of these businesses speaking to you. The fact is both of the businesses described could have been the best in their industries. However, if the culture is not congruent with the level of product you are providing, customers will not give you a chance.

The culture in your dental office should be the creation of an environment where the primary focus of every team member is serving your patients at the highest level possible. However, it is impossible for the quality of customer service to exceed the quality of the people who provide that service. Therefore, doctors must make the investment to properly and, more importantly, continually train team members to adopt and support the culture of the practice.

The secret to achieving a positive culture begins with every team member being "present." Everyone must set a goal every day to be 100% present in mind and body while striving to exceed your patients' expectations. This is why morning meetings are a must because they prepare your team to start the day focused and clear about their intentions while supporting the culture of the practice.

Here are a few examples centered on exceeding your patients' needs:

- Dental assistants escort the patient to the treatment room walking side-by-side side instead of five paces ahead.

- A team member remains in the treatment room while the patient is getting numb, building rapport, instead of retreating to the break room.

- Offer your patient a warm towel after their treatment and walk them out with a sincere and genuine "thank you."

- Follow up with a hand-written thank you note when patients refer new customers to your practice. Likewise, send a hand-written note welcoming new patients to your practice.

FLEXIBLE

It is essential that every team member is flexible, able to "go with the flow" without cracking under pressure. Dentistry is one of the few professions that operates on a strict schedule. We don't have the luxury of leaving our patient with a rubber dam on while we take a ten-minute coffee break because we are a little stressed out. There is no time in our schedule to go for a walk if you feel tired or, for that matter, even to take a phone call. Our patients depend on us to accomplish a certain task, in a certain amount of time, expecting the highest quality possible.

The treatment schedule is a living, breathing, frustrating thing that changes constantly. The most productive and successful practices are those that adapt to daily changes and keep their schedules productive. Changes in the schedule are a certainty, so all team members must accept this fact and adapt to those changes throughout the day.

I have seen team members actually become upset when a loyal patient is worked into the schedule with an emergency. What they are really saying is, *"I am inconvenienced."* They don't want to adapt to the needs of a patient who provides the practice with money and referrals—they want their needs to be first.

Who wants to keep a team member like that?

Flexibility should be a part of every team member's job description.

PROBLEM SOLVER

Anyone can complain, but it takes a great team member to not only address a challenge that exists in the practice, but also come up with a potential solution to that problem. It may not be the ultimate solution, but at least they are thinking beyond just complaining. Great team members find solutions to their challenges and don't expect someone else to fix those challenges for them.

I'm always amazed at what lengths people will go to avoid problems or setbacks. The reality is that problems are part of everyday life. Tony Robbins once told me that the day you don't have any problems in your life, is the day you are dead! So having problems is a really good thing.

A great team member doesn't look at a challenge as an inconvenience. They choose to look at it as an opportunity to come up with a new solution to make the practice better. If you want to be an invaluable team member, become a great problem solver.

RESPECTFUL

I think we all know the old adage, *"Treat people the way you want to be treated."* Unfortunately, in too many offices the environment or culture is so stressful and disorganized that team members don't always follow this rule of respect.

A great team member will always respect patients and fellow teammates. I have witnessed team members texting or reading magazines in the break room while their patient is forced to wait past their scheduled appointment time. How can you exhibit this kind of disrespect and then be at a loss as to why your patients don't accept your treatment plans or refer their family and friends to your practice? The message you are sending out is clear: Your time is more important than theirs. Being respectful means you value that person and you show this through your actions.

The Golden Age of dentistry is over. You can no longer just rent an office space, hang a dental sign, and expect patients to flock to your door and put up with disrespecting their time. If you choose, intentionally or unintentionally, to put patient needs second to your own personal needs, then expect your patients to find another more appreciative practice to join.

Great team members think consciously about what their patients must have gone through to get to your office on time. *They must have rushed to get the kids breakfast and off to school, hustled to a meeting at work, then snuck out early, and navigated heavy traffic, just so they could be ON TIME for their appointment.*

So how do you thank that patient for being on time? Don't make them wait for their appointment! After all they went through to get to your office, if they are kept waiting, the only thought running through their minds will be, *Why in the hell did I rush to get here?* Trust me, they will never make that kind of effort again.

I realize some of our colleagues in the medical field couldn't care less about making patients wait, but you have an opportunity to set your practice up for massive success if you just respect your patients by making it part of your culture to stay on time.

PROACTIVE

Don't you love being around people who just get things done? They seem to almost have extra hours in the day. You don't have to remind them every other day to finish what they said they would take care of last month; they just seem to get things done. They are proactive and self-starters that need little direction and less follow-up.

A great team member will handle issues that come up in the office without having to be told. They will fix things or make corrections when they see something out of line. Maybe it's organizing a more effective way to set up the instruments for treatment cases or discovering a more efficient way to ask for patient referrals or maybe even taking the schedule home to make confirmation calls for Monday's appointments. Now that's proactive.

Great team members set the example by not overlooking situations that someone else will have to deal with if they choose to look the other way.

BE AN EXPERT

Great team members strive to be the very best at what they do and seek out the necessary resources to make certain they are experts. Team members that consider themselves as experts don't wait until their doctor takes them to a continuing education seminar. They seek out education programs that will take their skills to the next level.

In many offices, the doctor is the only one considered an "expert," or lifetime student of continuing education. However, this can also be true for team members in any department. Your front office manager should be a master when it comes to dealing with patients' dental insurance, financial arrangements, and the never-ending management of the treatment schedule. Your dental assistant should know more about bonding restorations than most dentists, and your hygienist should have an in-depth knowledge of periodontal health and your soft tissue management protocol.

Doctors as leaders of their practices must set the example and create a culture that supports team members to be experts.

LAUGH, LIVE, AND CELEBRATE

Life is a journey, NOT a sprint or a destination. Surround yourself with people who appreciate their gift to be able to care for others, along with realizing the importance of life outside of the dental office. Dentists and their teams often find themselves in a sprint to build a practice, knock down debt, support a family, etc. ... They forget about laughing, living, and celebrating.

Dentistry is a demanding profession that challenges the mind and body equally. It is important that great team members celebrate both their successes and failures. Too often we discount successes and dwell far too much on our failures. Great team members acknowledge their failures with enthusiasm because they know they are learning something new and will grow from the experience. Great teams also take time to acknowledge their successes, as these are the results of having failed in the past—and having learned from it.

TEAM AGREEMENTS

*The best job goes to the person who can get it done without
passing the buck or coming back with excuses.*
—Napoleon Hill, author of *Think and Grow Rich*

At times, even great team members will have trouble working together. Someone will get their feelings hurt usually from a miscommunication or they might just be having an off-day. When tension among team members occurs, it can lead to an unhealthy culture in your practice. Team Agreements are a valuable tool to help your team operate together in a way that honors and respects each individual for his or her contributions to the practice and team.

Team Agreements are established to elevate the commitment of each person to the practice, creating a solid foundation for a high-performing team. The importance of knowing what each team member is responsible for eliminates the assumptions that a particular team member doesn't contribute as much as the others. This can commonly happen when no formal Team Agreements have been previously established. Team Agreements create a very special bond among people that will bring out the best in everyone.

Team Agreements are a verbal commitment to each other that removes assumptions and holds each team member accountable for his or her actions. They create trust and camaraderie that will move the entire team towards the goals and vision of your practice.

CREATING TEAM AGREEMENTS

SEE IT

Have your team think of characteristics that make up an outstanding team and list those specific traits for this imaginary dream team.

IDENTIFY WITH IT

Using the dream team list as the framework, ask members for up to five functions that they believe a great team performs that will move the team towards a specific goal. If, for example, they suggest "respect" and "good communication," then ask for specific interpersonal behaviors that produce respect and good communication among team members.

SIGN IT

Have each team member sign the document, which is their commitment to do their best to abide by the Team Agreements. This creates a public accountability and ownership of those agreements.

FRAME IT FOR ALL TO SEE

Great teams reach unbelievable success when they are in pursuit of the same vision or goal. Frame your Team Agreement and post it in the break room. This serves as a daily reminder about team members' commitments to each other and the practice.

TALK ABOUT IT

Talk about it, refer to it, and ask about it. Refer to your agreements when confronted with an action or behavior that is in violation of the agreement. Remind the person in violation by saying, "I thought we'd agreed to …"

EXAMPLE TEAM AGREEMENT

Communication: Agree to honest and open communication with all team members.

Gossip: Agree to not contribute to or tolerate gossip of any kind.

Support: Agree to provide support for all team members in achieving monthly goals and supporting the vision of the practice.

Listening: Agree to listen respectfully to the communication of others in order to understand their deepest meaning.

Resolve Problems Positively:

Agree to resolve problems, issues, and upsets with other team members directly and at the earliest opportunity. Avoid exaggeration and blame.

Performance:

Agree to constructively "evaluate results." The results of our teamwork will be measured against our predefined goals.

Integrity:

Agree to conduct yourself with high integrity inside and outside of the practice, always representing your team in a professional manner.

Conflict Resolution:

Agree to view all conflict as an opportunity to explore alternative views and different perceptions.

Team Meetings:

Agree to being on time, prepared, and open to contribute to morning and monthly team meetings.

Directness:

Agree to "say it like it is." Have the freedom to speak your opinions freely without judgment.

Leadership:

Agree to be a leader. Everyone is equally responsible for the effectiveness and success of the team. Agree to take responsibility for getting the job done while setting a positive example by showing leadership through honoring agreements.

Reliability:	Agree to "be reliable" and "present" for work every day, in a state to contribute and support the vision of the practice.
Be Open:	Agree to try new things. Be open to "try out" new skills or improved systems of the practice.
Learning:	Agree to look for opportunities and continue your education to become an expert in your field.
Creativity:	Agree to "think outside the box." Commit to creating new ideas that better support the team and the vision of the practice.
Health:	Agree to take care of yourself. Commit to good health, physically and emotionally, along with proper rest, and to avoid unnecessary fatigue and stress.
Celebration:	Agree to applaud individual efforts and recognize team accomplishments. Be specific and timely with positive feedback.
Fun:	Agree to enjoy the process, embrace your hard work, and HAVE FUN!

TEAM MEETINGS

*You gain strength, courage, and confidence by every experience
in which you really stop to look fear in the face.
You must do the thing you think you cannot do.*
—**Eleanor Roosevelt**

Team meetings seem to happen for one of two reasons: either to increase the productivity of the practice or out of sheer frustration when things are going terribly wrong.

Many dental offices seem to conduct their meetings with this type of hit-or-miss approach. The main reason for the inconsistency is that doctors consider these meetings "nonproductive" time. No money is being generated for the practice, and doctors would rather not pay their team members to sit around and complain, or listen to ideas that never will be implemented.

Regularly scheduled team meetings, especially at the start of each day, are essential to the success of your practice. Taking time to prepare for the day and review your goals is an invaluable tool to help serve your patients at the highest level.

Advanced preparation is the key to ensuring these meetings are productive and effective. If your meetings are disorganized and dysfunctional, then expect your team to follow suit. The true dynamics of a team can only be maximized when everyone is working together.

Productive team meetings help build and develop new relationships as a group. When you have the opportunity to hear and understand the individual challenges that each department faces day-to-day, you begin to find empathy for those challenges your teammates are dealing with. I think at one time or another we all are guilty of thinking we have the toughest job in the office, so it can be a humbling experience to understand and see things from a different perspective.

A culture where team members complain to each other during the day while diverting their attention from your most important asset, your patient, is a fast track to disaster. Your team needs to know there is a safe place where their voice can be heard, and team meetings can provide that refuge.

MORNING MEETINGS

Start your morning team meetings 15 to 20 minutes before your first patients are scheduled to arrive in your office. Gauge your time appropriately, so you have addressed everything for the day. Make sure your entire team is present and ready to greet the first patient when he or she walks through the door.

To begin your meetings, briefly review each patient of the day. Start by identifying the patients' scheduled and unscheduled treatments. Strategize how you will prepare your patient for the next step in their treatment plan. Review any special health history concerns or pre-medications they need to take before this appointment. Identify any special needs they may have, such as placing a towel under their head or not leaning back in the chair too far, and remember to thank them if they sent you a referral, or be sure to express your empathy with personal challenges they may have recently faced.

Reviewing the schedule in this way allows you to also discover pinch points in the day, such as getting to hygiene exams or saying "hello" to a perio-maintenance patient that doesn't necessarily need an exam. Preparation like this dramatically reduces the chance of getting off schedule and serves to remind your patients that **THEIR** time is more important than yours.

Morning meetings provide your team the opportunity to exceed patients' expectations. When your patients experience care that goes beyond clinical dentistry, they will naturally feel a bond with you and your practice. This is an example of the little things you must do consistently that will take your practice to the next level.

MONTHLY MEETINGS

This is a chance to celebrate with your team the many successes you have accomplished during the month. These meetings are more in-depth than morning meetings and provide you an opportunity to examine what you achieved and what you need to address in terms of personal and practice challenges. Monthly meetings provide team members a place to share their concerns, along with being recognized for an outstanding job.

These meetings are best held the first non-clinical day of the month. Friday usually is best, since most practices don't see patients on that day. With planning and preparation, these meetings should last no more than an hour or two. Give the appropriate time for each agenda item, but be aware of when it's time to move on.

Monthly meetings can be structured in any way that works best for you. Many practices, however, choose to begin by reviewing the previous month's production and collections numbers, new patients, attrition, team or patient challenges, and new technologies. Once the business portion of the meeting is completed, you have an opportunity for training sessions and *role-playing!*

All too often, we focus all of our energy on what our next marketing strategy is going to be or how we can incorporate a new instrument. Interestingly enough, we rarely seem to take the time to practice things such as case presentations, re-care enrollment, pre-scheduling, financial arrangements, and so on. If you are willing to get outside your comfort zone just a little, these exercises can be very rewarding.

Role-playing is an effective way to act out different practice scenarios, so that you can perfect your wording, sequence, and timing when speaking to patients. You can rehearse and make improvements to literally all of the practice productivity systems you have in place. Best of all, it's simple and fun to do.

Just pick a team member to act as the patient, get into character, and go! Try different ways to act out your presentations, and then allow time for every team member to give an opinion about how you did and how you can improve.

We often can't see our own shortfalls or simple ways to make critical improvements. It's almost impossible to make self-improvements when you're working with patients because you don't receive any direct feedback. Therefore, to get the most of your role-playing sessions, team members must be willing to play along without fear of embarrassment from anyone on the team. So put your ego aside, have fun, and start mastering all of your departments.

Role-playing is the fast track to reaching your goals.

ROLE-PLAYING EXAMPLES

- Case Presentations
- Treatment Plans
- Closing the Loop (review, praise, pre-frame)
- New Patient Experience
- Use of Intra-Oral Camera/ Incorporate into Hygiene & Restorative
- OSHA
- Chart Audit
- Scheduling
- Marketing
- X-rays Verbiage to Patients
- Soft-Tissue Management Protocol
- New Clinical Procedures
- Collections/ Financial Arrangements

Make a commitment to incorporate role-playing into your team meetings consistently and watch as your team soars to greatness.

MORNING TEAM MEETING

MAKE THIS AN OUTSTANDING DAY

Date: _____   Start time: _____

START EACH DAY WITH A PURPOSE & LIVE YOUR VISION

Be PREPARED to discuss each patient in detail.

The MORE we know, the BETTER we can SERVE our patients.

1. Review Previous Day's Production and Collection Numbers that Relate to Our Goal.

2. Review Scheduled Production for Today.

3. Review Each Patient's Name and Treatment Scheduled for that day.

4. Suggestions of Additional Treatment You Can Add to Today's Appointment

5. Review Medical History and Special Concerns

        a.   Allergies
        b.   Pt. doesn't like lying back, etc. …
        c.   High blood pressure

6. Review of Patients' History in the Practice

        a.   Completed treatment or treatment-in-progress
        b.   Treatment success/ complications
        c.   Note any pending treatment where you need to build VALUE.

7. State Any Referrals the Patient Has Given Us and Extend Them Special Recognition and Thank You.

8. Identify Potential Bottlenecks in the Schedule with Strategies for Solutions.

9. Identify When Hygiene Exams Will Be Completed for Each Hygiene Patient.

10. Review Progress Toward Bonus Goal.

11. Review Your Vision and Mission of the Practice.

MONTHLY TEAM MEETING

MAKE THIS AN OUTSTANDING DAY

Date: _____   Start time: _____

START EACH DAY WITH A PURPOSE & LIVE YOUR VISION

1. Review Month-End Numbers/ Practice Success Monitor
    a. Production
    b. Collections
    c. Dr. Production/ Hygiene Production
    d. New Patients
    e. Attrition

2. Compare Month-End Results to Goal & YTD from the Previous Year Using Your *Practice Success Monitor*

3. Identify & Discuss Areas of Success.

4. Identify & Discuss Areas of Challenges.

5. Review Marketing Efforts.

6. Review Calendar/ CE/ Vacation/ Days Off/ Staff Dental Day.

7. Discuss the Introduction of Any New Technology or Future Expansion Plans.

8. Role Playing/ Training Session.

OFFICE ENVIRONMENT

People become really quite remarkable
when they start thinking that they can do things.
When they believe in themselves, they have the first secret of success.
—**Norman Vincent Peale**

Have you ever walked into a restaurant and, based on the décor, made an instant judgment about the quality of its food? Of course you have. We all have. People make judgments or knee-jerk decisions like that every day. If I walk into a business and the furniture is dated or the interior is dirty, I assume it is behind the times or out of touch, so I'll probably leave. They might actually be amazing at what they do, but the environment is such a turnoff, I most likely wouldn't give them a chance.

People do the exact same thing when they enter a dental office. Believe it or not, a new patient will judge the quality of your practice based on the physical appearance both of the office and your team members.

Remember the days when the receptionist had a frosted glass window that would mysteriously slide open and a clipboard would appear with a voice, "Sign in," and then the window would slam shut! I always wondered who was back there and why they needed to hide. Most people have a certain level of anxiety when entering a dental office, so to help minimize patient fears and anxiety, dentists need to create a peaceful, soothing, and professional setting. So, I hope it goes without saying, the frosted glass window has to go!

Research indicates that you should give your office a mini facelift every four to five years. This could mean repainting the walls, replacing the window coverings, changing the artwork, or upgrading that old worn-out carpet to hardwood floors. However, the most important place to start creating your professional environment, so that your office reflects the quality of your work, is with cleanliness. I mean REALLY clean, smelling fresh and appearing clutter-free, especially in the areas you think no one notices. Have you ever reclined in your own dental chairs and looked at your ceiling? Your patients do everyday, and if they see cobwebs, they will naturally doubt the quality of care they are receiving. This is an absolute

MUST for every office, without exception.

Please throw away those old dental journals in your private office from the 1990s. You will never refer to them, and most likely the information is outdated anyway, so trash 'em. Toss anything that you have not used in the last year or two. For the hoarders among us, this might be difficult, but it's time to change your habits. A clean and organized office is a productive and profitable one.

Make sure that your practice signage and logo are professional and up-to-date. If your name is pealing off the front door, this will certainly present a negative image to your patients. Make certain the landscaping around your office is well-manicured, and your windows are professionally cleaned with all spider webs removed, inside and out.

Create an immediate and positive first impression by energizing the front entrance to your office. You can do this with lighting, painting the walls a modern color, especially removing all items around the entrance, so it feels open and inviting to patients. The reception room should be warm with fresh flowers or live plants, (please no plastic, Wal-Mart plants) light refreshments, soothing music, and comfortable chairs.

Treatment rooms should be the cleanest, most clutter-free spaces in your office. Find appropriate storage for supplies and instruments, instead of leaving them out on the countertops. Remember, our profession is intimidating enough to most patients, so keep this space free from distractions. Clutter equals disorganization, and disorganization equals a low quality of care in your patients' minds. The more instruments a patient can stare at, only makes them wonder if any of those will be used on them. Naturally this will increase their stress levels because, let's face it, they all look like they will hurt!

Restrooms … Need I say more? We have all been in public restrooms that are less than sanitary, which make us never want to return. Restrooms must be checked a few times per day to ensure they are clean. Make sure there are extra toilet paper rolls and a private place for feminine hygiene products. A supply of disposable toothbrushes and mouthwash is a nice touch, so your patients don't have to worry about knocking you over with their lunch breath.

The sterilization area must not only be clean, it must also look completely organized. Stacks of instruments out on the counter create uneasiness for your patients and, more importantly, your team. Team members want a clean, organized environment to not only work in, but if you want them to refer their friends and family, you can't have them thinking they would never have their personal dental needs cared for in your dirty office. They need to be proud of the office they are representing.

Patients are more informed than ever before, largely due to the Internet, so they expect to see updated office décor with modern dental equipment in your office. They are familiar with digital x-ray, lasers, intra-oral cameras, and, especially, modern dental chairs. If the white plastic covering on your delivery unit is beginning to turn yellow, then it might be time for an upgrade. These items are as much about marketing as they are high-tech equipment that increase the quality of care.

Creating a positive environment in your office is not a weekend project; it's a way of thinking and being. It must become part of the culture in your practice. A decorator can change the wall colors and choose the correct carpet and wall fixtures, but only you and your team can change the culture of your office. This means how you are dressed, your personal hygiene, your smile, etc. … Is your team in matching uniforms with nametags? Has everyone on the team had a recent hygiene and dental exam? Is everyone on the team pleased with his or her smile and proud to show it off to patients?

I have met doctors with smiles that were less than attractive, who could not understand why they were not doing more cosmetic cases. You need to be a living example of what you're offering to your patients. I have even heard some dentists say, *"If I make my office look really nice, my patients will think I'm charging too much."* The fact is your patients most likely already think you're charging too much, no matter what your office looks. Dr. Farran once told me that if dental treatment costs more than a pizza, most patients would think it's too much. The reality is, patients don't have a clue what dental care costs, so charge what you're worth and never make decisions out of fear or based on the unreasonable minority.

Remember, people are most interested in themselves, and what most people truly want is the best care for the lowest price. Who doesn't? I know I do. But I would not be willing to comprise my own dental care to save a few bucks and so will the majority of your patients. Stay true to the culture you have created in your office and watch your practice soar.

DR. MICHAEL DOLBY

SETTING GOALS

When I think of goals, the first thing that comes to mind is all the New Year's resolutions I've made during my life. I seem to think about my goals and say, *"This will be the year!"* Sadly, the year passes by, and only a few of my goals have been met.

I imagine that's an unfortunate scenario for most people. We all seem to believe that if we wish hard enough or allow enough time, our goals will be met. The reality is that life often interferes. Family and careers can dominate our time, and even with the best intentions, our goals have a tendency to fade away.

I vowed to end this cycle, so I began to research how other people were achieving their goals consistently. I found a 1979 study that involved the Harvard MBA program. This is a very competitive post-graduate program that accepts a mere 15% of applicants. The Harvard Business School interviewers asked new graduates a simple question: *"Have you set clear, written goals for your future and made plans to accomplish them?"* Surprisingly, only three percent of graduates answered, "Yes." Eighty-four percent of graduates had no specific goals while thirteen percent had goals; however, they were unwritten.

Ten years later, the same groups of MBA graduates were contacted to see how they were doing in their respective careers. The results were predictable. Incomes for the thirteen percent who had goals, but were unwritten, were twice as much as the eighty four percent who had no goals. The three percent, who had clear goals, wrote them down, and created a plan to achieve them, were earning ten times as much as anyone else in their graduating class!

Unfortunately, goals are rarely established in the majority of dental practices, and if a practice does set goals, they tend not to be reviewed or modified. I once asked a doctor what his production goal was for the year, and he responded, *"I'm not quite sure, but I think it's the same as last year."* It should be no surprise as to why this practice was struggling to grow.

WRITING DOWN YOUR GOALS

The Harvard MBA study demonstrates the benefits of establishing goals, writing them down, and creating a plan to achieve them. Writing down your goals causes you to FOCUS on that goal in a more thoughtful and concentrated way. The result is a clearly defined view of all issues related to achieving your goal. Remember, what you focus on, you tend to see, and then opportunities begin to show up. When you combine this with a specific plan to achieve those goals, and, more importantly, review and revise that plan, you are destined to accomplish that goal.

Another study, conducted by Virginia Tech professor Dave Kohl, found that eighty percent of Americans said they have no goals, sixteen percent said they have goals but don't write them down, four percent write down their goals, and, of those, only ONE percent regularly reviews the goals. His study confirmed that people who write down their goals earn nine times as much during their careers as people who don't write them down.

Dr. Gail Matthews, a psychology professor at the Dominican University of California, conducted a study that included 267 participants from a wide variety of businesses, organizations, and networking groups in the U.S. The results of her study were similar to the others with one addition: People who wrote down their goals, shared them with a friend, and sent weekly updates to that friend were 33 percent more successful in accomplishing their stated goals than those who merely formulated goals.

Based on these studies, we can predictably increase our chances of achieving our goals by doing the following:

- **Write your goals down** on paper.
- **Develop a plan to achieve your goals.**
- **Share your goals** with a friend and share updates.
- **Review your progress** consistently and **be willing to change your plan.**

So what goals should dentists create? There is not an "official" list of practice goals to follow. However, there are a few categories that successful practices share in common. It's more important that you establish goals that are first and foremost achievable for your team, but they should also challenge you a little each year, and it's critical your team clearly understands them.

Gross Production Goal:

This is the total amount of all revenue the practice produces in a year, based on your fee schedule. Calculate your yearly production goal by increasing the previous year's gross production number by, say, five or ten percent. You can also determine this goal by establishing what you would like to produce each day and multiplying that number by the number of days you will work in a year. Either way, the point is to clearly establish a goal and create a plan to achieve that goal. If you are starting a practice from scratch and you set a gross production goal of $1 million, you probably have set the bar a little too high. Your goal should be achievable and challenging at the same time.

Gross Collections Goal:

This number accounts for all the money the practice collects in a year. The number you chose for the gross production goal will obviously have an effect on this number; however, you want to aim for a goal of no less than 95 percent of total gross production. In other words, you will deposit 95 cents of every dollar produced in the practice. You might be thinking to yourself, *"Why can't my collection goal simply be 100 percent?"* This is a great question, and unfortunately you will have a certain amount of production that is just not collectable. For example, you most likely will have dental insurance contract write-offs that won't allow you to ask your patient for the difference between what their insurance paid for a certain procedure and your actual fee. You might also provide a discount if your patient pays in full at time of service, or you may donate treatment to a friend or family member. All of these scenarios will create uncollectable production.

It's important to remember the collection goal is an average number, so you might have one month where you collect 103 percent and another month where it is 95 percent. Don't panic if a particular month has a low percentage because more than likely the following month will be a greater number. Establishing a collection goal keeps you accountable for the production you have worked so hard to achieve. The success of any practice is based not on what you produced, but, more importantly, on what you collect and take home.

New Patient Goals:

Have you ever heard the phrase, *"If your business is not growing, it is dying"*? In fact, this is true for every business, including dentistry. Every practice needs a steady influx of new clients or patients in order to keep growing. It's inevitable your practice will lose patients for reasons that are sometimes out of your control. For example, patients will move, they change jobs, and unfortunately they even pass on. So every practice needs new patients to replace those who leave. Also, if you are maximizing your clinical efficiency, then at some point, your patient base will simply run out of treatment, so new patients will be needed in order for the growth of the practice to continue.

So how many new patients do you actually need? I tell audiences in my speaking engagements that a mass number of new patients is simply not needed each month to keep your practice growing. I can't stand it when I hear speakers at dental meetings bragging on how to attract 80 to 90 new patients per month. It would be impossible for me to properly service that many patients while delivering high-quality dentistry. The fact is that 10 to 20 high-quality, cash-paying, treatment-plan accepting, referral-giving new patients are far better than 80 to 90 patients who only accept the minimum treatment and then disappear, never referring a single patient to your practice.

Quality always beats quantity.

Monthly and Daily Production/ Collection Goals:

Great dental practices will break down the gross production and collection goals, so they can see a monthly and daily number. Sometimes looking at the overall goal number for the year seems almost fictitious because it's usually such a large number it's hard to determine how you're doing month-by-month or day-by-day. Breaking that number down to reflect a monthly, and then a daily, goal number can reduce it to a size that is easier to measure. This will allow you to precisely know whether you are moving towards or away from your goal, rather than waiting until the end of the quarter or year.

It is recommended to take this a step further by breaking down your goals into individual doctor- and hygiene-production goals. Determining what the doctor and hygiene departments need to produce on a monthly and daily basis will provide assurance that you will achieve your goal.

Please remember, it's important to set goals that are achievable. As I mentioned before, it is not reasonable to set a goal of one million in production the first year of a start-up practice when you have little to no patient base and no production history. The enthusiasm is great; it's just not reasonable. When setting goals for your practice, start by determining how many days per week you want to work. If you are starting from scratch, you will probably work five days per week, but for an established practice, you will most likely be practicing four days per week. However, some, that are ready to become incredibly efficient, will consider working three 10-hour days per week.

CREATING ACHIEVABLE GOALS

For the following example, I am making the assumption a dentist is working four days per week. When considering there are 365 days in the year, we will start by first subtracting the number of days we are not going to be in the office. Begin by eliminating all of the Saturdays and Sundays for a total of 104 days and, of course, Fridays for a total of 52. I'm also considering this dental practice will take off eight holidays, eight vacation days, and ten continuing education days throughout the year for a total of another 26 days out of the office. If we subtract the total of all the non-working days from the 365 days in a year, we are left with a total of 183 working days.

Now that we have decided how many days we will be in the office, it's very simple to determine what we need to produce each month to meet our goals. You can see from the table below that if our goal is to achieve $800,000 in gross production per year, we will need to have a monthly production number of $66,666, breaking this down to a daily production number of $4,371. You can even calculate this to an hourly practice production number of $546. With this detailed information in hand, you are now able to set achievable goals that you can monitor with accuracy.

SETTING GOALS

Practice Production Goal: $800,000
Daily Production Goal: $4,371
Monthly Production Goal: $66,666
4-day work week / 8-hour work day
Avg. 15.25 days per month

Example

365 possible working days

<104> Weekends

<52> Fridays

<8> Holidays

<8> Vacation days

<10> Continuing Education days

TOTAL Working Days: 183

Gross Production	Monthly Production	Daily	Hourly
$500,000	$41,666	$2,732	$341
$600,000	$50,000	$3,278	$409
$700,000	$58,333	$3,825	$478
$800,000	$66,666	$4,371	$546
$900,000	$75,000	$4,918	$614
$1,000,000	$83,333	$5,464	$683

OUTSTANDING CUSTOMER SERVICE

Everyone wants to be appreciated,
so if you appreciate someone, don't keep it a secret.
—**Mary Kay Ash, founder of Mary Kay Cosmetics**

In the fast-paced, automated, self-checkout, self-service, social media world we live in, it can feel as if customer service is dead. Although I think most businesses believe they offer outstanding customer service, my experience tells me that most do not understand what it means to provide a service that consistently exceeds a client's expectations.

So what is outstanding customer service in the dental office? Does it mean just being nice to patients, having a fancy office, or staying on time? According to Wikipedia, *"Customer service is a series of activities designed to enhance the level of customer satisfaction."* The key word in this definition is "enhance"—to *enhance* the level of satisfaction or, better yet, exceed that expectation.

Let's face it, the dental office can be a negative environment for a lot of people, and most patients are rarely excited about their upcoming appointments. Thanks to the Golden Age of Dentistry, where dentists, and even patients, expected the treatment to be uncomfortable, today's dentists and their teams must work extremely hard to overcome this negative stigma and strive to exceed patients' expectations. The good news is that we are really set up for success because customer service in healthcare is becoming scarce. Our physician colleagues have been bombarded with staggering patient loads that ultimately have created a strain on their ability to deliver virtually any form of customer service. It's not uncommon for a patient to arrive at a physician's office for a 9 a.m. appointment, wait until 10:00 a.m. or later to be taken to a treatment room where they sit alone, often in silence, and wait another 20 to 30 minutes for the doctor to arrive. With this kind of treatment, it would be hard for any patient to feel special.

If we define outstanding customer service as *"exceeding your patients' expectations,"* how can we accomplish this in our dental office?

The best example I can think of is from Walt Disney. He mastered the delivery of outstanding customer service and coined the phrase, *"Under-promise and over-deliver."* If you have ever been to Disneyland and got in line for a ride, you would see a sign that states the estimated wait-time for that ride. As you meander through the zigzag corral-type line on your way to the entrance, there are TV monitors promoting the ride you are about to experience. This is an amazing tool because it directs your focus on something other than how long you are actually waiting. To be absolutely certain they will exceed their customers' expectations, the listed wait-times for these rides are always exaggerated. So if the wait-time is listed as thirty minutes and you actually get on the ride in twenty, then naturally you are going to feel better about the wait. On the other hand, if the estimated wait-time is stated as the same thirty minutes and you end up waiting forty, you can be certain you are going to feel put out and disappointed.

There are many ways to apply this strategy in your practice. However, the delivery of outstanding customer service always starts with basic courtesy and common sense—treating people the way you would like to be treated.

As a whole, dentists tend to diagnose conservatively in fear of overwhelming their patients. This can be a dangerous path to go down because treatment can often change, as the case begins. When your patient is prepared for a simple filling but it develops into a crown that is more than three times the original estimate, your relationship and credibility are going to be strained, along with dramatically reducing your chances of even getting paid. Using the under-promise and over-deliver concept, it's important to diagnose the worst-case scenario, within reason, of course, so your patient is prepared emotionally and, more importantly, financially. If you set yourself up for success this way, there are no surprises or risk of damage to your relationship once the treatment is complete.

This philosophy can be applied to almost everything in your practice, including seating patients on time and finishing on time. I often hear dental teams boast about the amazing customer service they provide patients, only to witness them consistently running twenty to thirty minutes behind schedule.

So how do you really know if you are providing outstanding customer service? The answer is simple: Patients will show their approval by referring their family and friends to your practice. If you are finding that your existing patients are referring 75 to 80 percent of all new patients, you can be assured you are doing a great job of exceeding your patients' expectations.

I'm sure you can see that outstanding customer service is the LIFEBLOOD of any practice, so it's important to make this the central element in developing the culture of your office. Clearly, excellent clinical skills are not all that is required to build a great practice. Patients won't know how good you are until they know how much you care.

GREETING YOUR PATIENTS

I used to get my coffee at the same place every morning on my way to work, mainly because of its convenient location. The same person seemed to always take my order, and every morning he acted as if he had never seen me before. He never asked my name, could not remember what I drank, even though my order was the same every day, and didn't really seem to care that I chose his coffee shop over several others. It wasn't long before I started looking for another coffee stop to fulfill my morning addiction. The place I found has decent coffee, but its customer service is awesome. Every time I show up, they not only remember my name, they remember my drink and are always interested in what I'm up to. Even though their location is a little out of my way, I find myself wanting to be loyal to them because they make me feel welcome and appreciated.

It's so important to remember that our patients see us only a few times a year, so it is really a reunion for many of them. With the busyness of the office, seeing patients back-to-back and staying on schedule, the possibility to forget this fact and fall into the pattern of treating them as just another appointment is very real.

Ask yourself this: How would you greet a friend you have not seen in six months? Would you greet them with the words, "Next" or "The doctor is ready for you"? No, you would greet them by name and with a handshake and an enthusiastic smile.

Greet patients as if you are expecting them. It's really not hard to do since your day is run on a schedule and you know exactly who's coming in to see you. If you show patients that you are excited and appreciative to see them, it will set the stage for them to have a positive dental experience. When you treat your patients like friends, not someone who accidentally stumbled into your office, they will do the same for you through increased case acceptance and referrals of their friends and family.

You will hear me continue to preach throughout this book that the secret to a great practice is *"doing a lot of little things great, consistently,"* and greeting patients is definitely one of those little things.

STAYING ON TIME

When I first started in private practice, I went from seeing three to five patients per day, in dental school and in my general practice residency, to—what literally seemed like overnight—caring for twenty patients per day. My speed and proficiency did not allow me to keep up with the pace established by the previous dentist. I remember one particular day, late in the afternoon, I was running about thirty minutes behind schedule. Tired, frustrated, and defeated, I went to greet my last patient. Let's just say this patient was not the understanding type, and she was really upset with my tardiness. As I entered the room, to my surprise, she stood up, pointed her finger in my face, declaring, *"You picked the wrong person to be running late with!"* Obviously, this was not the highlight of my day. However, I learned a great lesson—the importance of a person's time—as well as a well-structured schedule with appropriate treatment times, designed so you can avoid getting behind and disrespecting your patient's valuable time.

Having to wait past scheduled appointment times is a consistent Top-10 patient complaint. I understand that sometimes this can't be avoided, but it certainly can't become the norm for your practice. When you schedule any appointment, essentially you and your patient are making an agreement to meet at a specific time and day to accomplish a particular procedure. So when you essentially break that agreement by making your patient wait, it only causes them to feel resentment. I've mentioned this before, but it's worth repeating—think about all your patient had to overcome to make it on time for the appointment. They most likely had meetings at work that needed to be adjusted, kids to get to school, or after-school events to deal with. The fact is, if your patients honor their parts of the agreement by showing up on time, it's critical that we show the same respect and see them on time.

I understand more than anyone that dentistry, with its rigid schedule, is more challenging than most other businesses that have flexibility throughout their days. With the majority of businesses, if a meeting runs long, most likely, no one is inconvenienced. However, in the dental profession, we have a specific task to complete within an even more specific timeframe, and when we fall behind from that schedule, many people are inconvenienced, and it can be almost impossible to recover that lost time.

Staying on schedule takes a complete team effort. You can set yourself up for success by monitoring treatment times and mastering clinical efficiency, which we will talk more about later. At the conclusion of every morning team meeting, you must emphasize the importance of honoring your patients by staying on time.

HAVE THEM AT "GOODBYE"

We all share patients. They move from one office to another, they move across town or out of state, their insurance plans change, or sadly, providers encourage them to change to a less-expensive office. Patients make changes regarding their health care providers that are the best fit for them, and unfortunately sometimes patients decide that your office is simply not for them.

This is an opportunity to step up and be a true professional whenever a patient leaves your practice. I have witnessed some incredibly rude responses from dentists who feel hurt when a patient decides to go elsewhere. That kind of reaction guarantees only one thing: Those patients will NEVER EVER return to your practice.

When a patient decides, for whatever reason, to leave your practice, it doesn't always mean forever. How you choose to handle that situation will determine if there is an opportunity in the future for them to return. First off, you must contact them with a personal phone call and thank them for giving you the opportunity to care for their dental needs. Then offer to transfer all of their records, free of charge, to wherever they choose. Let them know their new dentist can call you with any questions regarding the history of their oral health, and, most importantly, you want to let them know that if they ever want to return to your office, they are always welcome.

When you handle patient transfers in this type of professional manner, there is a good chance those patients one day will return to your practice. Have confidence that your customer service and quality of dentistry is so superior to any other office, that once the patient experiences inferior service, returning to your office is an easy decision. I have seen this many times over my career, and the amazing thing is that when a patient leaves your practice and you make it easy for them to return, they NEVER leave twice.

Commit to mastering outstanding customer service and exceeding your patients' expectations. Nothing you do will replace the value created when a patient knows you really care for them.

SYSTEMS

Practice Made Perfect
Blueprint for a Successful Dental Business

DR. MICHAEL DOLBY

BUSY DOESN'T EQUAL PROFITABLE

Most people are so busy knocking themselves out trying to do everything they think
they should do, they never get around to do what they want to do.
—Kathleen Winsor, author

One of the most common excuses I hear from dentists is that they feel the only barrier holding them back from success is simply more patients. We all need new patients to make our practices grow, but this is only one element in achieving a successful and profitable practice.

I attended one of the major dental meetings and stumbled onto a course where the speaker was bragging that his practice was seeing 50 to 100 new patients each month. My first thought was that it sounded like a prison sentence and exhausting! My second thought was that there was no way a single dentist could ever comprehensively take care of that many patients.

Unfortunately, this gross misconception encourages dentists to focus on attracting new patients rather than perfecting or introducing proven business systems to maximize the efficiency of their practice. Providing a superior dental experience is the best way to create long-term, stable growth in your practice.

The only way you can care for 50 to 100 new patients a month is to provide minimal treatment and/or a low quality of care. Remember: "Being busy does not equal being profitable." The only thing worse than being physically worn out after a long day, is being broke at the end of that long day too.

Let me ask you this question: Would you rather have a practice that had production numbers of $1.5 million per year with 80 percent overhead or a practice that produced $800,000 with an overhead of 57 percent? Some dentists bow down in front of doctors who boast about a $1.5 million production number and ignore doctors who produce only $800,000. If you truly understand that being busy doesn't equal being profitable, then the answer is easy. It's not about what you produce; it's about what you take home.

A practice with $1.5 million in production with 80 percent overhead is netting $300,000. However, the practice producing $800,000 with 57 percent overhead is netting $344,000. Why would you go to all the additional work and liability to produce another $700,000 in dentistry only to take home $44,000 LESS? The fact is—you wouldn't. When you completely understand the numbers and commit to working with maximum efficiency, you will reap greater rewards with less effort. That is how you create a highly productive practice with the least amount of stress.

You can have a very successful practice with just a few hundred patients, or even a million-dollar practice with 1,000 patients. You don't have to run from room to room, doing exam after exam, feeling out of control to have a successful and profitable practice. It is possible to have a practice where you spend quality time with each patient, at a pace that is steady and efficient, where you feel rewarded and fulfilled at the end of the day.

The key ingredient to achieving this type of practice is through the development and creation of a highly skilled and motivated team. You need a team with the focus, vision, and purpose to maximize the efficiency and profitability of your practice.

PRACTICE GROWTH SYSTEM

There is no scarcity of opportunity to make a living at what you love;
there's only a scarcity of resolve to make it happen."
—Dr. Wayne Dyer, psychotherapist

The Practice Growth System is a tool for you to have accountability of where your patients are currently in your practice. How often have you seen a new patient in your practice for an emergency exam, only to never see them again? It makes no sense to spend thousands of dollars on marketing to get patients in the front door, only to loose them out the back door.

Dental offices are no different from other businesses with multiple departments that handle customers. The successful dental practice model sets up a system consisting of five separate departments, each performing a specific function. To guarantee that your practice continues to grow, there should never be a time where patients (your customers) are not enrolled in one of these departments.

The five departments in the Practice Growth System are:

- New Patients
- Hygiene-Periodontal Care
- Restorative
- Re-Care
- Specialists

Each department is essential to building and growing your practice. It is critical that your patients remain as "active" patients, meaning they always have an appointment scheduled in one of the Practice Growth System departments.

As I mentioned before, you spend a great deal of time and money to market and promote your practice, internally and externally, with the primary objective of attracting new patients. The influx of these new patients is a critical element in the continual growth and success of your practice. Dentists can spend thousands of dollars on marketing campaigns that are successful and attract the type of patients they want. However, without a clear understanding of these departments, patients will end up on the broken-appointment list, usually never to be seen again.

Your team's primary responsibility is to strategically escort your patients through these different departments and have accountability for them at all times. When performed correctly, you will never find an exit point for any patient at any time.

New patients to your practice will most likely come from a personal referral or relocation, or in response to your marketing efforts. Once that patient schedules an appointment and arrives in your office, it is up to you and your team to make an unforgettable impression with your organization and professionalism while creating value for the services that you offer. The culture of your practice must be one where no patient leaves your office without an appointment in one of these departments.

Patients can enter the Practice Growth System in a number of different ways, but most begin in the Periodontal Care-Hygiene department or the Restorative department. From there, they may be referred to a specialist or transferred to Restorative Care for further treatment. For example, if they were referred to a periodontitis, they would reenter the Practice Growth System in the Periodontal Care department and possibly alternate Re-Care cycles with the specialist.

If your new patient went directly to the Restorative Care department, they would move next to the Periodontal Care department, followed by Re-Care. As you can see from the Practice Growth System graph, there never is an opportunity for patients to fall out of your practice.

I have evaluated numerous practices that are struggling to grow with thousands of patient charts and no idea of where these patients are in the practice. The Practice Growth System allows you to know exactly where your patients are at any given time, and it strategically returns them back into your system.

PRACTICE GROWTH SYSTEM

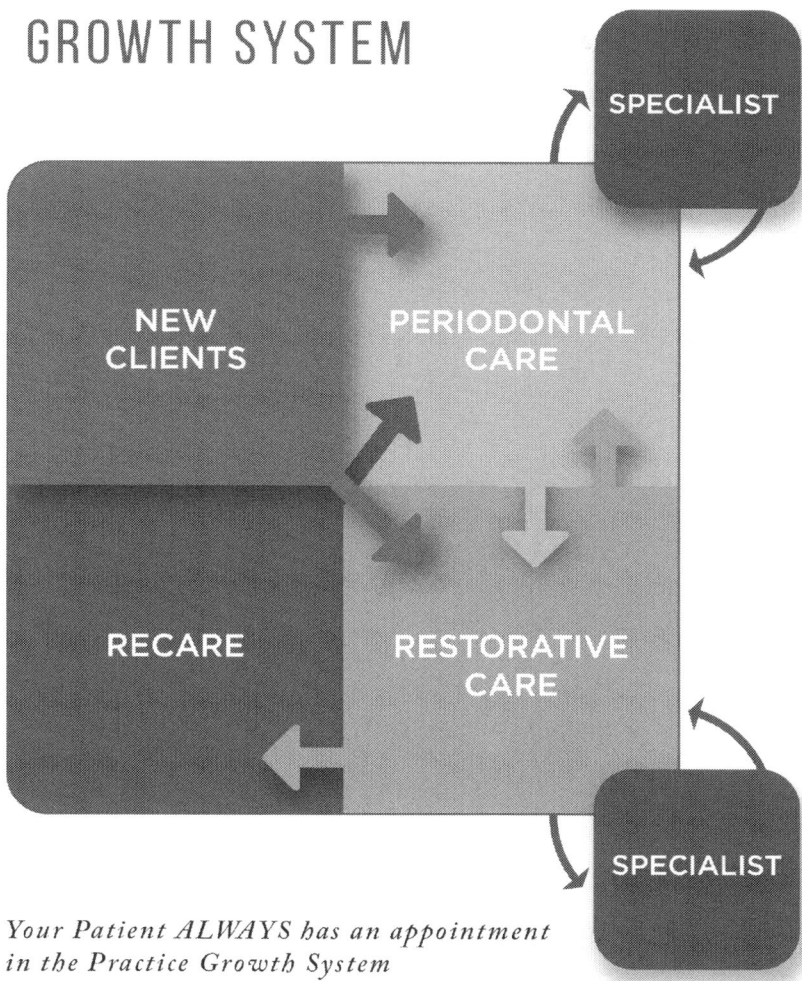

SPECIALIST

NEW CLIENTS

PERIODONTAL CARE

RECARE

RESTORATIVE CARE

SPECIALIST

Your Patient ALWAYS has an appointment in the Practice Growth System

CLOSING THE LOOP
(Review, Praise, Pre-Fame)

If people only knew how hard I work to gain my mastery,
it wouldn't seem so wonderful at all.
—Michelangelo

Closing the Loop is a business system that builds VALUE for the treatment you have completed or for the treatment you are proposing. When this system is used properly and consistently, it assures that correct communication between departments is not lost or misinterpreted, thus, increasing the value of your services in the minds of your patients.

How many times have you completed a new patient exam where you presented an amazing treatment plan and your patient seemed excited to get started, only to discover they left the office without scheduling an appointment? This is disappointing and frustrating; not to mention, this will severely hinder the growth and success of your practice.

When this happens, it's most likely due to the inability to create VALUE for the proposed treatment. The fact is, people will buy anything they value, even when they can't afford it. They will always find a way to get what they WANT and find excuses to put off the things they NEED when there's a lack of value.

As a patient is moved through the different departments in your practice, the effective transfer of information between team members is the first stage in building value for your services. When the doctor presents for a Re-Care or new patient examination, the hygienist must follow the script of *Review, Praise and Pre-Frame* and "close the loop" with the doctor, ensuring that no information is missed or misinterpreted.

The script begins with a simple REVIEW of what was found during the appointment. This may include what type of hygiene therapy was accomplished for that day, new treatment, proposed and/or pending treatment, along with any other special concerns.

We follow this up by giving PRAISE to the patient or letting them know what is going great for them. Mention a previous filling or crown that looks amazing; tell them their gum tissue looks better than ever; congratulate them if they quit smoking or have committed to flossing before bedtime. This step acknowledges what is working and what they are doing correctly.

PRE-FRAME is a review of any areas of concern and lets the patient know where they go next in their treatment plan. Patients look for direction from the doctor and team members, and it doesn't matter how big or small the treatment plan is. It must be broken down from highest to lowest priority, so your patient clearly understands the importance of where they are going next.

You can build value for the treatment plans you are presenting by following this script along with the strategy of creating urgency. Creating urgency simply stresses that the proposed treatment must be completed in a timely manner or it's possible the treatment plan will likely change. Most of the time you are presenting treatment plans to patients where they are completely unaware they had any problems because they are not experiencing any discomfort, so this is all new information for them.

It's important to remember that patients don't know what they don't know, so it's our responsibility as their dentists to motivate and educate them, so they can make informed decisions. For example, if you have diagnosed a crown, from a large, broken-down silver filling with unsupported tooth structure, and if they decide to wait to begin their treatment, they might be facing a root canal or even an extraction when they finally decide to start.

The highest value for the services you offer occurs when your patient is in your office, especially if there is no discomfort. As soon as they leave your office, the value essentially goes away. After all, it doesn't hurt, so it's out of sight and out of mind. If your patient fails to schedule an appointment while they are in your office, your next opportunity to address this might have to wait six months when they return for their hygiene exam. So it's critical to create this urgency before their treatment plan changes to a more expensive, and possibly more difficult, restoration.

It is critical to break down the treatment plan according to the highest priority, or your patient has a good chance of becoming overwhelmed by the amount of work that has been proposed. When patients are overwhelmed with a large treatment plan, this leads to confusion;

confusion leads to decreased value; and decreased value leads to not scheduling their treatment.

Strive to use your own words when going through the *Review, Praise, and Pre-Frame* script. I'm not a fan of pre-scripted words because they sound fake and insincere. Use words your patients can understand, not dental jargon like MODs, buccal pits, and lingual cusps. This will do nothing to increase the value of your treatment plan and will only leave your patients wondering what you were talking about. Speak in a language that non-dental people can understand.

The process of *Closing the Loop* accomplishes two important things: It builds value for what you accomplished that day, along with the treatment you are proposing.

Example of
"Closing the Loop"

Review: *Review what you accomplished today with the patient there listening.*

Doctor, today for Mary, we completed an oral cancer-screening exam and found no significant findings, and completed her perio-maint cleaning. Her gum tissue looks great and pockets are within acceptable limits. I have to say, the re-care schedule she is on is really keeping her mouth in optimum health.

Praise: *Give praise to something the patient is doing that is good.*

Doctor, I wanted to let you know that Mary is doing a great job flossing and using her waterpik before she goes to bed every night. Also, the onlay you did on the lower right looks and feels great to her.

Pre-Frame: *Review any areas of concern and where you want to go next.*

Doctor, we have some treatment that was diagnosed at her last visit, and, as you can see from the intra-oral photos, it appears the upper left may be getting worse. I would also like you to check the upper right first molar because it looks like there may be a cavity starting under her crown.

RECEPTION

*People who soar are those who refuse to sit back
and wish things would change.*
—**Charles R. Swindoll, author and pastor**

The word "reception" means to greet or welcome. This should be the culture
that is experienced by every patient that enters your office. However,
sometimes this can get lost among the day-to-day busyness and shuffling
of patients in and out of the practice.

The reception desk can sometimes be referred to as the central command
post of your office. This is where the majority of calls are answered, the
schedule is battled here everyday, appointments are made and sometimes
rescheduled, financial arrangements are secured, and, most importantly,
this is the entry point for every patient that visits your practice. There is
not a more important department in your office because if you can't shine
here, most patients won't give you another chance.

In our world today, any new patient can get a general feel for your office by
simply visiting your web site. There they can see the doctor's credentials,
usually photos of the team members, any specialty training, and the
number of years you have been in practice. However, the most likely
determining factor for a new patient deciding to remain in your practice
is based on how you make them feel when they enter your reception room.

In fact, as I have said previously, new patients will initially judge the quality
of your dental care based entirely on their experience of how they are
received in your office. Patients will ask themselves the questions: Are you
approachable? Are you organized? Are your team members friendly? And,
most important, do you seem happy they are in your office as a new patient?

Often this position is not given the proper consideration it deserves. I
would be extremely careful and choose a special person for this position
that is not only multi-talented but can build rapport easily with people,
so you can be assured that every patient has a positive experience in your
office.

DR. MICHAEL DOLBY

OFFICE MANAGER
The Quarterback

I think we all can understand the importance of the quarterback on a football team. This is the person that is held to a slightly higher set of standards, and teammates tend to rely on this person's talents to carry the team to victory. The quarterback must perform under pressure, and their tenacity will likely determine whether the game ends in a win or a loss.

Your office manager could be considered your team's quarterback. The leadership and organizational skills required for this position are critical to the long-term success of your practice. They manage an ever-changing treatment schedule, answer phones, check patients in and out of the practice, make financial arrangements, and handle the never-ending dental insurance challenges. They keep the day flowing, patients happy, and the practice productive.

I have witnessed a so-called office manager reading *People* magazine at her desk during the middle of the day. Considering this is the busiest department in the office, I found it odd as to how this person was finding enough downtime to read a magazine. When I asked the doctor why they chose this person, they went on to tell me that she has been in dentistry for over 20 years and knows everything about how to manage a dental office. I can assure you I have never met a superstar office manager that finds time to read magazines at his or her desk. However, the likely fact is, this person knows very little about how to run a dental office, but unfortunately it's probably more than the doctor!

Many doctors put their trust in the hands of a single person they call their office manager because they are either intimidated about learning how to properly run their business or they are simply too busy learning new skills as a dentist. Either way, if you choose not to personally manage your business and lead your team, your fate will be in the hands of someone else that has a lot less to lose than you do as the owner of the business. I can't stress enough the importance of educating yourself regarding the practice management skills necessary to not only manage your business but, more importantly, become the leader your practice needs. This will allow you to then introduce an outstanding office manager to the practice, and together you will make certain your practice and team are always moving towards your goals.

I have seen some amazing office managers come from non-dental backgrounds, so don't be afraid that they don't have any so-called previous dental experience. I always recommend hiring people that already have the skills you can't teach them, like being nice, courteous, sincere, a team player, genuine, etc. When you interview a new team member and you instantly like their personality, trust me, your patients will too. You can teach a person with a great personality to operated Dentrix or how to file an insurance claim, but you can't teach them to be nice and have people like them. These are the most important skills that will have the biggest impact on your practice. So make a well-considered decision when choosing this critical member of your team.

GREETING PATIENTS
Friends

It's a great feeling to run into a friend whom you haven't seen in years. Don't you find yourself instantly happy, feeling close, and connected to that person? If you bump into an acquaintance and they remember your name, family, and what sports your kids are playing, you can't help but like that person, even if you really don't know them that well. So ask yourself, how do you greet patients in your office that you haven't seen in six months?

As we discussed about outstanding customer service, I've witnessed team members greeting patients with the words "Next!" or "The doctor is ready for you." Then they proceed to walk three paces ahead of the patient as they are shown to the treatment room. Would anybody consider this a warm greeting? Can you really expect patients to feel valued or appreciated with this kind of reception? Your patients see you, on average, two or three times a year. To them, it's a reunion. Unfortunately, with the stress of running a busy office, they often get treated as just another patient.

It's an ABSOLUTE MUST that ALL team members treat your patients like friends!

Your office has the advantage of knowing who's coming in and at what time. You know their first names, and you should have notes on their interests or what they were up to the last time they were in your office. With all of this information, you are already set up for success.

DR. MICHAEL DOLBY

When a patient arrives, greet them like a long-lost friend. Extend a handshake or, if it's appropriate, a hug. Always address them by the name they prefer. For most people, this will be their first name. However, the older generation may prefer Mr. or Mrs. followed by their last name.

Make the greeting personal. Make certain to look the patient in the eye and let them know how much you appreciate their coming to see you. Remember, the quickest way to build rapport with someone is to make the conversation entirely about him or her. People love to talk about themselves, their kids, or anything that is going on in their lives.

Your patients have more dentists to choose from than ever before, and they chose YOU!

Team members should escort every patient to the treatment room by walking side-by-side and strive to never leave them alone in the treatment room with nothing to do. Sitting alone in a room can only make the minutes seem like hours, and nothing will upset people more than having to wait. If there is going to be a delay until treatment begins, this is an excellent time to have a team member stay in the treatment room and build rapport with your patient. You can find out what is happening in their life or inform them about the advances in cosmetic dentistry and specialty services you offer. Ask them how they want their smile to look in the next five years. Get the conversation flowing, and you might be surprised at what you find out.

ANSWERING THE PHONES
Have them at "Hello"

Answering the office phone is an opportunity to make an amazing first impression. However, the opportunity is often missed because team members usually have no formal training as to the correct way to accomplish this task.

I prefer a system of guidelines that allow team members to answer the phone in a natural, unscripted manner. It's important to remember the person on the other end of the call wants to be a patient in your practice or they wouldn't be calling, so treat them with respect and enthusiasm.

Patients will respond with the same amount of enthusiasm and excitement as you present to them, so it's important to use powerful words such as *terrific, great, wonderful,* and *awesome*.

Although the front office receptionist or office manager will usually answer the majority of phone calls, everyone on the team should be trained and willing to take on this important task.

FIVE RULES FOR ANSWERING THE PHONE

(1) **Always pause a moment before answering the phone.**

No one likes to hear that someone is out of breath.
This only gives the impression that you are too busy or, worse,
disorganized to accommodate new patients and deliver
outstanding customer service.

(2) **Answer on the third ring, MAX.**

No excuses. This is a team responsibility.

(3) **Have a consistent response.**

*"It's a GREAT DAY. Thank you for calling Cottonwood Creek
Dental. This is Sherry. How may I help you?"*

If a team member is not available, reply:
*"Cynthia is not available. Is their anything I can help you with
today?"*

(4) **Always ask if you can assist the caller.**

Remember, the caller is looking for results, so do your best to
accommodate them.

(5) **Take a message.**

Follow the message format, so nothing is missed. The easiest way
to implement this system is to provide a message pad at each
phone station. It's important to take down the date of the call,
the person's name, the message, a return phone number, and the
best time to call.

Shopping Fees

You will often get calls from potential patients who are simply shopping fees. Many practices ignore these people and assume that they are just cheapskates, but think about it for a moment from the patient's perspective. They probably don't have a relationship with a dentist or they wouldn't be calling you, and, more importantly, they don't realize that all dentistry is not created equal. In their mind, a crown is a crown, so it's natural that price becomes the only way to choose one dentist over another. It doesn't mean the person is a bad patient; it just means they need to be educated as to the quality and craftsmanship of different restorations, and this is your opportunity to do so.

When speaking with potential patients who are asking about fees, be sure to quote basic prices. Let the person know that no two teeth are the same and no two crowns are the same. For an accurate quote, offer to see this person for a complimentary evaluation.

Team Member: Thank you for calling Cottonwood Creek Dental. This is Cynthia. How may I help you?

Patient: I was calling to see how much your crowns are?

Team Member: I'm so glad you called us. We use one of the best dental laboratories, so we can be sure that our patients are getting the highest-quality crowns. Our crowns start at $989, and I would be happy to offer you a complimentary evaluation by Dr. Dolby, so we can provide you with an exact cost. Will you be using any dental benefits?"

Patient: Yes, I have Delta Dental through Micron.

Team Member: That's wonderful. Many of our patients work there, and our new patient coordinator, Sherry, is very familiar with Delta Dental Benefits. I have an opening in Dr. Dolby's schedule at 10:30 on Thursday morning. Will that work for you?

This is just how simple and easy it can be to build value for your services, even with people who are shopping prices over the phone. This certainly beats the office that quotes their fee and then allows the patient to say,

"Okay," and hangs up. Provide yourself the opportunity to enroll every patient who calls into your practice.

With enthusiasm, invite EVERY patient to join your practice.

NEW PATIENT FORMAT

Have you ever had a friend recommend you try out a certain business because they had such an amazing experience and for whatever reason the service you received was marginal at best? While another friend of yours tried that same business at a different time and had a great experience? This happens when businesses do not have formal systems to follow that ensure all customers have the same experience.

In the dental office, when every team member follows the same format when interacting with patients, you can be certain that every patient referred to you will have the same outstanding experience as the next.

(1)   **Greet your patient with a warm welcome.**
a.   Shake the patient's hand and use their name.
b.   Build rapport.
   i. Where are they from, referral source, look for things you have in common.
c.   Discover chief complaint.
   (reason for coming to the office)
d.   Show before and after pictures, or other promotional material to support your patient's concerns.

(2)   **Patient Information Forms**
a.   Medical history
b.   New patient form
c.   HIPPA forms
d.   Financial policy form

(3)   **Pre-Op Findings**
a. Blood pressure recording
b. Oral cancer screening
c. Take FMX or Panorex x-ray and any additional images of concern.

c. Chart areas of concern.

d. Take intra-oral photos of at least four areas *(good or bad)*.

e. Periodontal probings (PSR)

f. Study models *(for cosmetic or comprehensive cases)*.

(4) **Hygiene**
a. Complete Prophy, Debridement, or RP
b. Finish appointment with a warm, scented towel

(5) **Doctor Exam**
a. Display the four intra-oral pictures.
b. "Close the Loop" (Review, Praise, Pre-frame).
* Debbie did awesome today. We completed her oral cancer exam with no findings. We measured her pockets, and her gum tissue is in great shape. She is doing a great job with her flossing, and her gums look better than ever. She has a crack in a sliver filling on the upper right that we will need to correct before it breaks further. We discussed the importance of flossing at bedtime, and we currently have her on a four-month re-care schedule.

(6) **Dismiss Patient**
a. Escort patient to front office and "close the loop" with receptionist and/ or office manager.
b. Shake the patient's hand, use their name, and thank them for coming in today. Let the patient know you look forward to seeing them at their next appointment.

MANAGING THE SCHEDULE

Taming the Monster

One of the most important jobs of the front office is to manage the treatment schedule. This is an ever-changing, breathing, eating, time-consuming monster that your front office team must conquer EVERY DAY. Anyone who has ever managed a dental treatment schedule will tell you that at the end of the day, one minute after all the confirmation calls have been made, the phone will ring with a change request in the schedule.

The team member who takes on this job must be flexible, patient, and willing to go to battle with the schedule no matter what the day brings. The treatment schedule is the life blood of the practice since it contains all the production for each day, so if there are holes or gaps with unproductive treatment time, this will dramatically affect whether the practice is profitable or not.

Reminder Postcards

Postcards are still a great way to remind patients that their hygiene appointments are just around the corner. These cards are hand-addressed by the patient at the end of their hygiene appointment, and the theory is that they will recognize their own handwriting and not assume the postcard is junk mail. The reality is that most people will need more than this, so I also rely on personal confirmation calls to make sure certain patients will arrive in my office on time.

Confirmation Calls

Good old-fashioned customer service seems to be disappearing in America, and I believe the majority of people want it back. When was the last time a business treated you as if you were important? Self-checkout seems to be taking over almost every business, so we rarely need to speak to anyone unless an "error" message pops up on the scanner. How do you get connected and feel loyal to a business when they eliminate all human interaction?

Automated patient reminder systems are becoming more common. These services contact your patient base via e-mail, text, or phone to remind them of their appointment. This type of automation can relieve some of your team's workload, but there can be a potential downside. This type of service with a computer voice can be viewed as annoying by some patients and may actually hurt your practice more than it helps.

Personal confirmation calls are needed to continue the culture of outstanding customer service in your practice and to assure your schedule remains a productive one. Calls should be made 24 to 48 hours before your patient's appointment, and, yes, the appointment is not considered confirmed until you speak to the person. Taking time to speak to your patient accomplishes two things: It allows you to review and build value for their scheduled appointment, and it provides an opportunity to answer any of your patient's questions.

Here is an example of effective scripting for personal confirmation calls:

"Hi. This is Cynthia, and I am calling to let you know that Dr. Dolby is excited to see you at your 2 p.m. appointment tomorrow. He was wondering if you had any questions or concerns that he could address."

When you confirm appointments this way, patients won't feel as if you are being a pest by reminding them of their appointments. On the contrary, they will feel as if you are concerned with their well-being, which builds more value and less short-notice cancelations.

The dental profession is an intimate and, at the same time, intimidating place for the majority of people, so providing customer service that is personal is absolutely necessary if you want your practice to grow.

Priority Short Notice List

Creating a priority short notice list will help in managing a productive treatment schedule. This is a list of patients who are available to come to your practice on short notice and fill those precious voids that develop in your schedule during the day.

When you schedule a patient for their next treatment, ask if they would like to be placed on the priority short notice list if an earlier appointment opens up. Make sure they can get to your office within 20 to 30 minutes, so if you do call them at the last minute they can actually fill the void in your schedule.

Productive Scheduling

Nothing is worse than running off schedule. In order for a treatment schedule to stay on time and be productive, the first priority is to determine accurate treatment times.

You can imagine that inaccurate treatment times would only create an inefficient, chaotic office. Your team may seem busy, but the practice will not be profitable. A schedule with appointments that are either too short or too long will create a stressful day.

In the majority of dental practices, the dentist often determines treatment times, but from my experience, they are the wrong person to decide this. Let's just say that dentists seem to be overly optimistic about how long treatment procedures really take them, while the team members tend to judge more accurately.

One way to determine the correct treatment times is to keep a running log of simply how long procedures take. Instruct your dental assistant to record these times, and after one month you will see an average time for multiple procedures. You can use these numbers to accurately schedule your appointment times. Repeat this process at least once a year, and possibly two or three times a year if you have been in practice less than five years, until your scheduled treatment times equal your actual treatment times.

Your goal is not to be the quickest dentist, but strive to be the most efficient while maintaining the highest quality of care. I will discuss it further when I address clinical efficiency, but proper organization, preparation, and knowing where you are going with a treatment can drastically reduce your current amount of chair time.

PROACTIVE HYGIENE

*The best and most beautiful things in the world
cannot be seen or even touched.
They must be felt with the heart.*
—Helen Keller

I have found that the majority of successful dental practices focuses attention primarily on the productivity and efficiency of the hygiene department. When you stop and think about it, this is where all the diagnosis, treatment planning, and production dollars are generated, so naturally this should be a department of focus. Consider the hygiene department the engine that keeps your practice moving forward. Without a strong hygiene department and clear systems to support that department, a practice is heading nowhere but to a slow death. Remember: If you're not growing, you're dying.

Amazingly enough, I've watched doctors treat the hygiene department as an inconvenience because they have to break away from their operative procedures to perform hygiene exams. Your hygiene department is the only other generator of production in your practice, so it makes sense to focus on this department and find the absolute best team members to fill these roles. In fact, I repeatedly hear from hygienists the frustrations they feel when they diagnose root planning or promote the use of laser therapy, but then their doctor will downplay their diagnosis, especially if it's a friend, and tell the patient all they need to do is floss more! Now put yourself in the place of the hygienist that just spent an hour building rapport and value for the scaling and root planning your patient desperately needs, only to be deflated with absolutely no support from the doctor.

When practices have no formal hygiene department systems in place, the hygienists are often left to figure things out for themselves, and over time without the support of the dentist, it's not long before they end up doing one bloody prophy after another, simply because—if the doctor doesn't seem to care, why should they? Meanwhile the practice struggles to figure out why the hygiene department and the operative schedule are not as productive as they should be.

During tough economic times, practices often panic and look to the hygiene department as the best place to start cutting costs. That's like not putting gas in your car to save money and then wondering why it doesn't run! It drives me crazy when I see the hygiene hours in a practice reduced in an attempt to avoid paying the hygienist's high wage. The doctor ends up performing all of the cleanings, which is the quickest way to sabotage a practice.

If your practice is experiencing challenges within the hygiene schedule's productivity, shift your focus to the unscheduled appointment list and reactivate patients back into the re-care system. That is far more productive than devising a strategy to avoid paying for a hygienist and transferring that job to the dentist.

Two major problems arise when a dentist takes on the hygienist duties: There tends to be less concern with actively diagnosing periodontal disease along with building the hygiene department, and, as a result, there is less time for restorative work. This strategy quickly gets out of hand, even if implemented for the short term. If you're going to wait for the hygiene schedule to fill up, you will find mysteriously that never seems to happen.

Proactive hygiene means creating a culture in your practice where there is as much concern for treating periodontal disease as there is for a 10-unit veneer case. The cosmetic cases may be more exciting, but you will never find one in your schedule if you don't focus on growing your hygiene department. Remember, this the source for the majority of your restorative production.

You can start by building half-days into your hygiene schedule and then expand from there. Do your best to sequence your hygiene schedule, so there is little if no downtime between patients. There's nothing worse than having your hygienist make confirmation calls or file charts because there is a 30-minute gap until their next patient. Build the best, most condensed day possible and if that turns out to be a half-day, fine, no problem. I would rather send my hygienist home after a productive half-day, than have them in the office all day for a half-day's worth of work.

Proactive Hygiene Provides

* Treatment Opportunities
* Patients with Optimum Oral Health
* Referrals of their Family and Friends

Everyone on your team must adopt the system of addressing and treating periodontal issues. This can range from simple gingivitis to advanced periodontal disease. Without a system of precise steps, consistency in this department will be lost. Dentists have a duty to offer patients the best treatment opportunities available, and this includes periodontal care.

There are many ways to treat periodontal disease and an equal number of opinions about which treatment is best. Studies consistently report that 50 to 75 percent of people in the United States suffer from some type of periodontal disease. Therefore, this suggests that most practices are simply not diagnosing or treating gum disease. Maybe this is why the highest appointment failure rate is in the hygiene department. Creating value creates retention, and if you and your team don't value hygiene care, then why would you expect your patients to feel differently?

Most people realize they need their teeth professionally cleaned at least twice a year, but many feel if they brush and occasionally floss and, more importantly, they are not experiencing any discomfort, they assume everything is fine. So when another opportunity comes up that conflicts with their scheduled hygiene appointment, they will choose the alternative because there is little to no value for the "cleaning."

The Proactive Hygiene System creates consistency in your diagnosis and treatment planning and that leads to an increase in value for your hygiene services.

PROACTIVE HYGIENE
Goal

Each hygiene examination will include the following procedures and information:

DR. MICHAEL DOLBY

- Early detection, diagnosis, and treatment of periodontal disease for <u>ALL</u> patients.

- Complete hard and soft tissue hygiene examination.

- Note all defective restorations and/or decay present. It's either broke or it's not. Commit to eliminate, *"Let's put a watch on this,"* from your vocabulary. Find more in the chapter on *Confrontational Tolerance.*

- Use the Diagnodent on all teeth along with an explanation of this technology and build VALUE.

- Explorer test: Feel the root surfaces for any rough or irregular areas. If positive debris is found with bleeding, regardless of pocket depth, quad scaling is indicated.

- PSR probing: Complete a PSR probing once a year on all patients and continue with a full mouth probing if quad scaling is determined.

- Take a minimum of four intra-oral photos of potential restorative treatment areas to show to your patient. Always include a pre-op and post-op picture of the lower anterior tartar buildup. This one really builds the value.

Educate, Inform, Build Rapport!

DEFINITIONS OF PROACTIVE PERIODONTAL CARE

<u>Prophy:</u>   Light buildup. No bleeding. Light supra-gingival scaling followed by rubber cup polishing.

Re-care: 6-month.

<u>Debridement:</u>   Moderate buildup. Very slight bleeding and light calculus. Mainly supra-gingival with some sub-

gingival scaling followed by rubber cup polishing. Fine scale 2–3 weeks after debridement, with specified laser therapy if needed.

Re-care 4–6 months.

Quad Scaling: Moderate-severe buildup. Moderate-severe bleeding. Quad scaling, laser therapy, and/ or the use of chemotherapeutics. Perio exam and periodontal maintenance in 3–4 months. Patient is ALWAYS a perio-maint. patient.

Re-care: 3–4 months, based on patient's home care.

SOFT TISSUE MANAGEMENT PROTOCOL

TYPE 1

Gingivitis: Gingiva pink, firm, healthy tissue. 3–4 mm. pockets. *(possible localized areas of minimal 4 mm. pockets)* Minimal buildup, no bleeding.

Treatment: Adult prophy   Re-care: 6–month

TYPE 2

Advanced Gingivitis: Inflammation of the gums characterized by changes in color, form, position, surface appearance, and presence of bleeding and/ or exudates, tenderness upon probing, bad breath or bad taste, probing depths of 3–5 mm. with areas of little to no bleeding.

Treatment: Debridement with possible laser therapy
                    Re-care: 4–6 months

TYPE 3

Early Periodontitis: Light generalized or only localized heavy calculus. Progression of the gum inflammation into the deeper periodontal structures and bone, with slight bone loss, pocket depth 4–5 mm. with slight loss of connective tissue attachment and possible, slight loss of bone on x-ray. Bleeding present.

Treatment: Debridement/ laser therapy
                    Re-care: 2–4 months

TYPE 4

Moderate to Severe Periodontitis: Presence of generalized moderate to heavy calculus. Progression of the gum inflammation into the deeper periodontal structures and bone, with slight to severe bone loss, gingival recession, pocket depth 5–6+ mm. with loss of connective tissue attachment and possible tooth mobility.

Treatment: Quad scaling/ laser therapy
                    Re-care: 3–4 months

RECARE SYSTEM

No person was ever honored for what he received.
Honor has been the reward for what he gave.
—**Calvin Coolidge**

When we consider the value of a patient, often the only measure we find ourselves using is the amount of money a patient has actually spent in our office. While there is some truth to this way of thinking, a more business-minded approach would take this a step further. Instead of only looking at the dollar amount that a patient has spent in your office, we must also consider how many patients that person has referred to the practice. I think you will be amazed when you discover just how much income can be generated to the practice from just one patient, without their actually having spent a lot on dentistry themselves.

If a patient walks into your office, pays cash for a ten-unit veneer case, and never returns, then this patient really has only temporary value to your practice. It's great to get that influx of new income, but the true value of a patient is measured over time. When patients promote your practice to their friends and families, the value generated here is far greater than any one-time veneer case.

A properly managed re-care system produces far better oral health and restorative care for your patients regarding the dentistry you have already completed. It also allows for the diagnosis of future dentistry and motivates patients to refer other people to your practice. Your re-care system is the source for accumulating active and, more importantly, referring patients in your practice. It is essential to the growth of your hygiene department and cannot be overlooked.

Dentists spend thousands of dollars each year on marketing campaigns for the sole purpose of attracting new patients. When the marketing efforts begin to pay off and new patients start coming through the front door for treatment, your team must rely on the Practice Growth System to keep these patients' statuses as "active" in your practice, meaning they are seen in your practice a minimum two times per year and are working towards completing their treatment plans.

Your new patients must remain in one of the departments in the Practice Growth System, so they are not lost and end up on the unscheduled appointment list. If your team does not make the re-care system a priority, the only thing growing in your practice will be unproductive voids in your schedule.

Your goal is to NEVER let any of your patients fall out of your re-care system.

A dental "guarantee" is a great strategy to keep patients as active members in your re-care system. After completing any procedure, inform your patient that you will provide a guarantee for the restorative work you have just completed for up to two years if they remain current with their re-care periodontal therapy. When dentists have the opportunity to keep a close eye on the restorations during a patient's re-care exam, they most likely will notice any complications that may arise and have the opportunity to correct them with ease. However, if they only see these patients every four or five years, instead of a quick repair, the restorations will most likely have to be completely replaced.

So the next time your front office team member is confirming appointments and your patient wants to cancel, they can gently be reminded that their $1,100 crown they just completed will unfortunately be out of warranty. This is called "leverage," and you will be surprised by how many patients change their minds and keep their scheduled appointments once they realize their warranties will expire. The reality is that you will use your common sense and good judgment for every restoration you have completed that pre-maturely fails and needs replacement. If a restoration breaks or a crown comes off, you most likely would correct that problem free of charge anyway, so a warranty is simply an incentive for your patients to keep their scheduled re-care appointments.

Every patient MUST schedule their next re-care visit before they leave your office. The typical re-care patient will schedule out at least six months plus one or two weeks to allow for flexibility and not risk compromise to their dental insurance benefit. If your patients hesitate to schedule, create urgency by letting them know that your schedule fills up quickly and you want to make sure there is an appointment time available for them that works best in their schedule. You can always offer to change their appointment if needed, but this will keep them as active patients in your Practice Growth System.

This strategy will assure patients are not lost in the pages of your unscheduled appointment list.

When you are reactivating a patient who has been out of the re-care schedule for more than six months, first attempt to work them back into the hygiene schedule, whether there is pending restorative treatment or not. Depending on how long it has been since you have seen them, more than likely the pending treatment will have changed anyway. In order to create VALUE for your services, remind them of the great progress they have made with their oral health and tell them you don't want to loose any of those gains. Reactivating patients back into the hygiene department will allow you a face-to-face, more personal opportunity to build rapport and value for the pending treatment they still need to complete.

You can see how a Pro-Active Re-Care System is essential to the long-term growth and success of your practice. Your team must make this a priority in your practice to create VALUE for this service, so your patients will honor their re-care appointments.

REACTIVATION SCRIPTS

Hygiene

"Good evening, this is Carolyn at Dr. Dolby's office. How are you? I am calling today because Dr. Dolby is really concerned that he has not seen you since February and wanted to make sure that the fillings you have on your treatment plan don't become worse. So I'm calling to see what is the best day and time that works in your schedule to have your teeth examined and cleaned."

Pending Treatment

"Good evening, this is Carolyn at Dr. Dolby's office. How are you? I am calling today because Dr. Dolby was very concerned that he has not seen you to take care of your cavity that he found back in January, and he's worried that it may

be getting worse. I'm calling to see what is the best day and time that works in your schedule to get that fixed before you start to feel pain."

Remember, that for most of the treatment you diagnose, your patients will not be currently experiencing any pain, so essentially it's out of sight … out of mind. All the more reason to remind them they still have these cavities, and they will and do get worse.

3 STAGES OF CLINICAL EFFICIENCY

Tolerance is giving to every other human being
every right that you claim for yourself.
—**Robert Green Ingersoll, political speechwriter**

I remember, back in dental school, how frustrating and complicated it was learning to do my first treatment of any kind on a live person. My heart was beating, sweat was building up on my forehead, and it was hard to get my hands to stop shaking. G. V. Blacks' preparation guidelines were firing away in my head, and my drill-sergeant instructor was hovering over my shoulder to make this an experience I would never forget.

I'm sure all dentists have gone through something like this during their early years. However, with time and practice, what used to seem impossible is now accomplished with relative ease. What I find interesting, though, is that for many dentists it takes approximately the same amount of time to prepare a crown now as it did just a few years out of dental school. Rational thinking would suggest treatment times would significantly decrease with the more proficient we become, but this rarely seems to be the case.

If you ask most doctors how much time they allow in their schedule for a typical crown preparation, the usual response is about an hour. However, if you ask their dental assistant or scheduling coordinator, they will give a much different answer, almost certainly longer. The truth is, rarely is there focus on improving the organization and efficiency of our clinical procedures. This lack of clinical efficiency keeps many dentists from maximizing their productivity goals.

Clinical efficiency defines the productivity and efficiency of your treatment procedures. If it takes 40 minutes to complete a high-quality crown restoration, the benefits of profitability and patient satisfaction are greater than if that same crown takes two hours to complete.

When your schedule allows an hour for a crown preparation and the patient walks out the door an hour and a half later, it creates a chain reaction. You most likely have another patient in the reception room that has been waiting for thirty minutes, a hygienist who is upset because her patient has been waiting for their exam, and a dental assistant who is frustrated because she doesn't have time to turn over her room. Your crown patient also is late for a meeting and has no time to stop at the front desk to pay. Sounds productive, doesn't it?

3 STAGES OF CLINICAL EFFICIENCY

Focus

Organization

Knowing Your Outcome

Focus

As I described in *"Becoming a Great Team Member,"* what we focus on, we can create. Our primary goal is focusing our attention on becoming the most efficient and productive with every dental procedure we perform, while maintaining the highest quality of care. When you direct your attention and focus to mastering this part of your practice, this is the first step in providing your patients with the best dental experience possible—along with removing the unnecessary stress that clouds the culture of many dental practices.

Organization

Having your dental assistant run to the next room because something you seem to always need is not in the instrument setup or sorting through a pile of unnecessary instruments is no way to prepare for a smooth appointment and will sabotage your chances of mastering clinical efficiency. When you are unorganized, it creates chaos, and chaos causes a stressful environment in your treatment room. Creating an efficient clinical setup for every procedure you do is the first step to mastering clinical efficiency.

First, decide the absolute minimum amount of instruments you need to complete each procedure. We all have instruments sitting in our tray setups that never get used, but we keep placing them back into the setup because that is what we have always done. Be realistic. Do not include instruments that you "might" need or only need on rare occasions. You can always grab those instruments as needed. Instead, plan for the everyday, routine procedures, which includes your gauze, cotton rolls, anesthetic, etc. Then arrange these items in the order that you will use them. This will allow you to quickly move through the procedure without searching for anything on your treatment tray.

Your clinical setup should be minimal, clean, and organized, with everything ready for you to begin treatment. Take a picture of each setup and include these in your employee handbook, so that any new team member will know exactly how to set up your rooms correctly. Remember to keep it simple and plan for a stress-free appointment.

KNOWING YOUR OUTCOME

All great artists have one thing in common: They begin a painting with the end in mind. They can see the picture long before the first brushstroke ever hits the canvas. You can imagine this allows them to move through their creative process smoothly, and, more importantly, they know when they have reached the end.

This phase of clinical efficiency is where most dentists will be able to dramatically improve their clinical procedure times. Often a dentist struggles with improving in this area because they begin procedures with no picture in their mind of the final result. Even more critical, there is not a clear plan or system in place to follow regarding how they will complete the treatment. When there is no clear vision of what the end product looks like, the results will be "puttering"—hoping the perfect margins magically show up—and unfortunately what ends up determining the completion of the treatment is that they simply run out of their scheduled appointment time.

Before every procedure, have a very clear picture of what you are trying to accomplish by running through the steps in your head and visualizing yourself at every step until the treatment is complete. Be clear in your mind about what the perfect preparation, impression, and temporary will look like. Visualize all of the margins, clear and distinct with a highly polished temporary, seated all before the end of the scheduled appointment time.

I have seen some of the top cosmetic dentists break away from their patient in the middle of the procedure, to get a clear picture in their heads of what they were trying to accomplish. Don't think this visualization strategy is just for rookies. The best of the best do this with almost every case they take on.

MASTERING CLINICAL EFFICIENCY

Crown/ Onlay Preparation

(1) Greet your patient, build rapport, and explain their treatment to increase the *value* of your service.

(2) Give anesthetic *(SLOWLY—you won't hurt people this way).*
   (a) While anesthetic is taking effect:
      Make temporary form
      Take pre-op pictures
      Choose shade and complete lab slip
      Take opposing arch impression (if necessary)
      Complete hygiene check if necessary

(3) Prepare teeth/ buildups, etc.

(4) Take post-prep pictures.

(5) Begin temporary.

(6) Take impression.

(7) Trim temporary while impression is setting up.

(8) Seat temporary.

(9) Show patient before and after pictures *(building even more value).*

(10) Escort patient to the front desk and "close the loop."

HYGIENE NEW PATIENT EXAM

(1) Greet patient by their first name, shake their hand, welcome them to your practice, and build rapport.

(2) Review patient info, health history, any chief complaints.

(3) Take necessary x-rays.

(4) Hygiene Exam—pocket depths, restorative options, etc.

(5) Hygiene procedure—prophy, debridement, quad scaling, while educating at-home hygiene and the co-diagnoses of restorative recommendations.

(6) Dr. exam—"Close the Loop."

(7) Pre-schedule/ Re-Care.

(8) Escort patient to front office—"Close the Loop."

CONFRONTATIONAL TOLERANCE

I once heard Greg Stanley present the term, *"confrontational tolerance,"* referring to the low level of tolerance regarding a person's ability to confront difficult or sensitive situations. I believe this is the single most common behavior that keeps most dentists from reaching their professional goals: They find it difficult to tolerate the sensitive situations that result from revealing to patients the true state of their poor dental health.

Entering my 20th year of practice, I have never had a patient overjoyed after being told they have a dental treatment that needs to be completed. I see young dentists and hygienists right out of school, with all the enthusiasm and ambition in the world, excited to begin their careers. They could not be happier when they find decay under a crown or advanced periodontal disease that warrants four quadrants of root planning. They are so excited to share their professional knowledge with anticipation of their patient's appreciation for what they discovered. Unfortunately, this enthusiasm quickly disappears as a result of their patient's negative response to their diagnosis. Over time this response can become deep seeded in the dentist, thus slowly allowing confrontational tolerance to get the best of them. Without even thinking, they begin limiting their diagnosis to what they believe their patient will accept—downplaying obvious dental breakdown as if they are not sure what to do and instructing their dental assistant to put a "watch" on it!

Not disclosing a full and complete treatment plan to our patients is not only absurd, it's unethical and unfair. The exact person, your patient, whom you are "protecting" from being upset or disappointed, would never understand why in the world you would only tell them a portion of what needs correcting, regarding their dental health. Presenting only what you think the patient will accept is entirely about your own inability to deal with a confrontation.

Ask yourself if you have ever been in this situation: It's the end of a crazy busy day, you're tired, and you are called for your last exam. This particular patient you already know likes to challenge everything you diagnose. You see a small cavity, but you try to convince yourself it might just be a stain. You tell yourself it probably won't be the end of the world if it's not corrected now and choose to take the "non-confrontational path," telling your patient that everything looks good, or, worse, you fall back on the *"We will put a watch on it"* excuse.

This is the exact sequence of how dentists allow confrontational tolerance to get the best of them. If this avoidance or lack of confrontation is not addressed, it has the ability to cripple or destroy your practice. Your team will quickly pick up on the fact that you only diagnose what you think patients can afford or, worse, can handle hearing, and this will lead to internal conflicts among your team. Team members want to know that patients in the practice are being cared for exactly the same way they themselves would want to be cared for. So when that level of professionalism is compromised, so is the integrity and culture of the practice.

Remove the term "watch" from you dental vocabulary. This term serves no one and only takes you further away from mastering confrontational tolerance. When you think about it, what are we watching? Cavities will continue to grow, so you can either watch that process happen or you can inform your patient. They may not be happy—who would be?—but they certainly don't want you to tell them everything looks fine when it clearly doesn't.

A tooth is either broken or not. If it's broken, then it needs to be fixed. Don't compromise a person's opportunity to have their dental health corrected because you want to avoid their disappointment. Trust me, no one will ever be delighted they have a cavity, so get over trying to protect them from being disappointed—it's not going to happen. Every patient, whether they are the first or the last of the day, deserves the same professional, high-quality care, diagnosis, and treatment presentation. No exceptions.

When you have made the commitment to master confrontational tolerance and always provide full comprehensive exams, there is nothing more powerful than when a patient calls your office with a toothache, and you inform them that you already had that tooth diagnosed in their treatment plan. Your patient will have no doubt that you truly know what you are doing, and respect will fill the room. However, if you had not previously addressed that tooth and your patient calls, they will be disappointed as to why you missed this and wonder even more what else you have overlooked.

To break this pattern, you must commit to the belief of when you charge a patient for a complete exam, you must give them just that, a complete and through exam. You must commit to presenting EVERYTHING you see that will improve their oral health, even if you know they will not be thrilled with the news.

The culture of your practice must be one that is always about preserving your patients' rights to choose whether they complete their dental treatments or not. Commit to never withholding anything that you would correct in your own mouth. This starts with comprehensively diagnosing and presenting that exact diagnosis with enthusiasm. Don't ever let confrontational tolerance take control of you or your practice.

TREATMENT OPPORTUNITIES

There is no question that plenty of dental practices have been affected by the last downturn in the economy. Unfortunately many dentists have chosen to use this as an easy excuse to why their practice is not more successful while others are quick to point blame on too much competition. The truth is, in any economy, well-managed practices with established business systems, combined with leadership, seem to experience little or no financial setbacks during these so-called tough economic times. Why? They are not only well managed, but, more importantly, they know where to find treatment and maximize those opportunities.

When the schedule has openings or the practice just isn't as busy as it used to be, many dentists believe that all they really need to solve this problem is more new patients. So they rush out and invest in expensive marketing campaigns with billboards, newspaper and magazine ads, social media campaigns, and maybe even TV. What they don't know is that as much as every practice needs a steady influx of new patients, those new patients won't solve any of their financial woes unless the systems within the practice are changed.

There are more dental treatment opportunities today than ever before. While the introduction of fluoride has dramatically decreased the vast amount of decay, there is still plenty out there that needs addressing—you just have to look for it. When I first started in private practice, what used to be a stain in the groove of a tooth is now a full blow cavity. These cavities are subtle and are not going to be detected using the old school "stick-your-explorer in-the-hole" test. They need a more advanced tool, such as the Diagnodent or illumination, so you can actually see the decay sitting directly under the enamel shell. I can't tell you how many times I have removed just the top layer of enamel of what appeared to be a dark stain, and a black hole appeared that wasn't evident on the x-ray; however, it went 4 mm. into the tooth before the decay was completely removed! Cavities only need an access point in either a crack or separation of an old restoration, and the bacteria will grow like crazy when it reaches the dentin. On the surface, this may not look like much, but this is disease that needs to be corrected.

Have you ever experienced a new patient that has transferred to your office, where they tell you they are current with their cleanings at their previous office, and you end up diagnosing a substantial amount of dental work? How does this happen? Maybe the patient is exaggerating about the accuracy of staying true to their re-care appointments, or their previous dentist simply wasn't completing exams. Far too many offices make the crucial mistake of failing to address the thousands of dollars of dentistry that comes through their office daily.

Baby boomers are supplying the dental profession with an abundance of silver fillings that are 10–20 years old and are all most likely in the failing stages. Let's face it, wherever you are on the amalgam debate, it's a known fact that mercury will expand and contract as it reacts to hot and cold temperatures, just like a thermometer, so when it contracts and the margin pulls away from the tooth, an access point is created for bacteria. When the mercury expands, a crack can happen either in the tooth or in the filling itself, creating again an access point for bacteria to begin growing below the enamel. The fact is, tooth-colored fillings are what your market wants, so this can be the perfect opportunity to replace an outdated silver restoration with something the patient actually wants.

Every dental office has an abundance of similar treatment opportunities that are either simply overlooked or ignored because *"It's only a buccal pit"* or *"It's just a stain."* This is confrontational tolerance creeping in, so you tell yourself, *"It seems okay for now."* Commit to identifying these subtle cavities and educate your patients as to what is really happening with their teeth. Intra-oral photos are a great way to show them exactly what the cavity looks like and to build value for the treatment you are proposing.

I spoke previously about the power of focus and the phenomenon of what we focus on we have a tendency to see. Have you ever attended a continuing education class on "veneers," and you were so fired up about doing this type of dentistry that when you returned home, it seemed that out of nowhere veneer cases started showing up in your office? The fact is, those veneer cases or treatment opportunities were always there, but because you just started focusing on veneers, that's what you started seeing. So if you want more treatment opportunities—it starts with sharpening your focus.

The bread and butter of most practices in the United States is centered on general dentistry. Even the top cosmetic dental offices will only generate about 25–30% of their revenue from strictly elective or cosmetic work. That leaves 70–75% of revenue from crowns, fillings, dentures, hygiene, etc. Look for the little things like one- and two-surface fillings, incisal chips, abrasion areas, and dark stains, as much as the big stuff, like crowns, bridges, and implants. A quadrant of composite fillings can be extremely profitable, especially when you have mastered clinical efficiency.

We have yet to mention probably your largest treatment opportunity, which is the previously diagnosed treatment in your patients' charts! Yes, the abundance of treatment that has yet to be completed. Instead of investing in elaborate marketing campaigns, direct your efforts to the thousands of dollars that are just sitting in your patients' charts ready to be scheduled. When you think about it, this should be the easiest treatment to get on the schedule because these people already have a relationship with your office and they know that something needs to be done, so all you need to do is create the value for that treatment.

Now that you are committed to diagnosing even the little things, I'm going to teach you what comprehensive diagnosis really looks like.

COMPREHENSIVE DIAGNOSIS

Comprehensive diagnosis could also be named "*mastering confrontational tolerance,*" as we have discussed previously. Comprehensive diagnosis simply means diagnosing everything that is required to bring your patients' oral health to optimum levels, pain-free with no decay. It's funny how this was exactly our intention when we left dental school, but somewhere in our careers a change occurred, and before you knew it, the definition of comprehensive diagnosis became whatever you felt the patient could handle hearing.

We have all heard the phrase, *"Diagnose as if it were your family,"* which is fine. However, in such a situation, confrontational tolerance never seems to creep in because your family tends to accept everything you suggest when it's FREE! In the real world, you are presenting treatment plans that are time-consuming and expensive, so some patients will react with frustration and disappointment. After a few years of this uncomfortable confrontation and rejection, some dentists will naturally shy away from this and stop diagnosing multiple units or complex cases in fear of the reactions from their patients. Now I'm sure many dentists will read this and say to themselves, *"That certainly isn't me."* However, what they don't realize is this avoidance happens so slowly that over time most dentists don't even understand this is a problem. They might be aware the production numbers are down and the practice is not as busy as it has been in the past, but they won't associate this with a lack of diagnosing and will quickly link this lull in the practice to a bad economy or increased competition.

ASKING PERMISSION

The easiest way to avoid falling into this trap is to start your exams by asking permission. Yes, asking permission. What I mean by this is after you have done an amazing job building rapport and before you recline your patient back in the chair to begin your clinical exam, ask them if it's okay for you to inform them about everything in their mouth that potentially could be a problem or already is problematic. Most dental problems are "out of sight, out of mind" for the majority of people and we never really know what level of care new patients to your practice have previously experienced. I'm consistently amazed when a new patient tells me they just had a complete exam 6 months ago and $5,000 worth of dentistry is staring right at me! The importance of asking permission and informing them of what you are doing is to educate your patients on the level of care you provide. Far too many dentists just recline their patients back in the chair and simply tell them *"let's take a look"* without ever inviting them to be part of the process.

In 20 years of practice, I have never had a patient say no to this question. Not one patient has ever said to me, *"Doc, can you just tell me the things that are really bad?"* Let's face it, no one really wants to have any dental work done if they can help it, but they certainly don't want to have a broken tooth or an infection surprise them. So, it's critical, prior to our examination, that we encourage each patient to have an open mind to everything it will take to get their mouth the healthiest it can be.

When you start your examinations this way, your patient will feel as if you are on their side. More importantly, they don't feel as if you are diagnosing things just to make your next car payment. It's important to set yourself up as their personal liaison and partner before you ever begin presenting them with any treatment you've discovered.

FORECASTING

The next step to mastering comprehensive diagnosis and defeating confrontation tolerance is through what I call "forecasting." This is a strategy I use daily, so that I will never be tempted to withhold or minimize a diagnosis from a patient, no matter how uncomfortable it seems at the time. For example, a new patient comes to your office and talks about how amazing their previous dentist was and how much they appreciated his or her gentle touch. During your clinical evaluation, you discover the reason for this dentist's gentle touch was because they hadn't actually been touching the patient's teeth at all, as evidenced by the advanced periodontal disease. In this situation, it's natural to feel apprehensive knowing you have to inform this patient they have essentially been neglected while they thought they had been receiving great care.

How I prepare myself for this situation is that I first acknowledge internally the uneasiness I may be feeling about presenting my treatment plan. I then "forecast" in my mind the discomfort of withholding or minimizing my diagnosis in fear of their rejection or unhappiness, and try to determine if that discomfort is greater than the pain of having to tell them in the future that they need a root canal, perio-surgery, or worse—an extraction! We all know that dental decay grows, and these problems will only get worse. So when it comes time to present any treatment plan to a patient, imagine what it will be like if you DON'T present your comprehensive diagnosis. A few years later, they may be losing their teeth, and, all the while, you had been telling them that everything was fine! For me, this type of pain surpasses all others. I would much rather present my comprehensive diagnosis, deal with their short-term unhappiness, and rely on building rapport, assuring them that I am on their side and committed to correcting this problem.

DIAGNOSE EVERYTHING

Have you ever made the mistake of judging someone's ability to afford restoring their smile based on the way they look or how they dress? I have, and boy was I ever wrong. A gentleman once arrived in my office unshaven, poorly dressed, and very soft-spoken. My first impression was that he didn't have a dime to his name, and this would be a charity case at best if I chose to take it on. He said he was getting married and wanted a new smile. I agreed to evaluate him, and after a comprehensive evaluation, I presented the ideal treatment plan without fear of confrontational tolerance. I diagnosed eight maxillary and eight mandibular veneers for a total of about $15,000. I expected him to walk out the door, but, instead, he reached into his pocket and gave us $5,000 in cash as a down payment to reserve his appointment time. I later found out that he had been a farmer his entire life and owned thousands of acres that he had just sold to a housing developer for millions. The lesson I learned from that experience has never left me to this day. I am most thankful that I had the courage to stay true to my comprehensive diagnosis and not diagnose based on what I had thought he could afford or what he could handle hearing.

STEPS TO COMPREHENSIVE DIAGNOSIS

Ask Permission

Forecasting

Diagnose Everything

DR. MICHAEL DOLBY

FOUR STAGES OF EFFECTIVE CASE PRESENTATION

Once you have mastered comprehensive diagnosis, there can be a tendency to provide too much detailed information on everything the patient needs that usually results in blank stares. Too much information leads to confusion, confusion leads to doubt, and doubt leads to not scheduling. People will never value something they don't understand. Treatment plans that are presented in Latin rarely create value. Patients don't know anything about MOD, RPD, endo, etc., so avoid creating confusion with language your patients cannot understand.

"Mrs. Jones, you have a large cavity under your crown on the upper right. Your crown must be replaced a soon as possible, or you risk a root canal or, worse, losing the tooth all together."

We know that patients won't buy anything they don't value, so what really is the best way to get your patient to see the value of your treatment plan? And what is the best way to motivate them, so they will schedule this treatment? The answer is "rapport." In order for any treatment to be accepted by your patient, you must first be in rapport. When you are in rapport, you can move through your case presentations efficiently and expect a positive outcome. If you are not in rapport and attempt to present your treatment plan based solely on the fact it needs to be done, you most likely will be confronted with endless questions and indecisiveness. This leads to uncertainty, and uncertainty leads to not scheduling.

Once you are in rapport, the delivery of your comprehensive diagnosis must be presented with absolute certainty. Your verbal and nonverbal communication must be decisive and to the point. Nobody wants a doctor to give suggestions for their treatment and then ask them to decide on their own. Dentists have all the education, and your patients rely on that education to help you make the best treatment decision for them.

THE PRESENTATION TRIANGLE

Presenting your comprehensive diagnosis to your patient face-to-face is essential to a positive outcome. You cannot effectively communicate without eye contact, but unfortunately this is how treatment plans are presented in far too many dental offices. The dentist usually sits behind the patient and talks to the hygienist or dental assistant, making reference to the computer screen or the patient's chart. There is very little or no interaction with the actual patient sitting in the chair, and the dentist wonders why they have trouble getting their patients to schedule their treatments.

The Presentation Triangle is a tool that will ensure your patient is part of the process when you are presenting your comprehensive diagnosis. The goal is to present clearly, decisively, and with absolute certainty. You must first believe in the treatment you are proposing and that it is the best choice for this particular situation. If you present your plan in an indecisive and ho-hum manner, don't expect your patient to be motivated enough to schedule with you. Patients have a million and one things they would rather do than spend the afternoon in your office, so it's crucial they understand and associate VALUE with the treatment presented.

The Presentation Triangle arranges the doctor and hygienist in front of the patient during the treatment presentation. This alignment allows the hygienist to "close the loop" with the dentist while including the patient in the conversation. The patient has the opportunity, while sitting upright, to hear what was accomplished during their visit and the concerns that were discovered. The doctor can refer to the intra-oral pictures on the computer screen in front of the patient, building even more value for the treatment recommendations. When you present your comprehensive diagnosis in this manner, your patients will feel like they are part of the decision process and never feel like outsiders. This is their treatment plan that is very personal for them, so making them the center of the presentation is critical.

FOUR STAGES OF EFFECTIVE CASE PRESENTATIONS

Problem

Effective case presentations have four distinct stages, and the first step is to present the "problem." This is simply stating what is wrong with a particular tooth. It may be a defective restoration, decay, a fracture, etc. We want to let the patient know why this tooth is compromised and, more importantly, why it needs to be corrected.

Solution

Next, we present the "solution" to that problem. You can explain what materials and procedures you will use that will produce an amazing result to correct their problem. In most cases, you will have the opportunity to present a solution that is superior to what they had before. For example, replacing a silver filling with a bonded composite filling certainly is a superior restoration from the patient's point of view because they are changing out a black filling for a white one!

Consequences

After you present the solution to their problem, it's critical for you to inform your patient of the "consequences" of not completing the recommended pending treatment, that it could always allow the cavity to get larger or more expensive and turn into a root canal or even an extraction. It's very important your patient knows what can and will likely happen if this treatment is delayed. Most patients won't have any pain associated with your proposed diagnosis, and since it's out of sight and out of mind, they must understand this situation can and will get worse over time.

Urgency

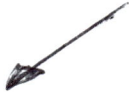

The consequences of delaying treatment lead us to the last stage, which is building "urgency." Since most people don't want to be faced with a root canal or a tooth extraction, they will choose to follow your recommendation and schedule their treatment. However, without creating some sense of urgency, patients will tend to fall back on *"If it doesn't hurt, then it couldn't be that bad"* reasoning.

Patients need you to give them a timeline to have this recommended treatment completed. When I hear doctors say to patients, *"Get in as soon as you can,"* what this tells the patient is they have time and it's not that serious. Because if it was serious, they assume you would have given them more specific timelines of having this completed. Let's face it, all of our lives are busy, and even though your patient may have great intentions of having this treatment completed in the next few weeks, life's schedules creep in, and before you know it, a few months have passed. I like to create in my mind what this tooth will look like in six to nine months and create the urgency based on that scenario because if treatment is delayed, this is exactly what it will look like.

STOP TALKING

I have seen doctors do an amazing job building rapport, comprehensively diagnose, give an effective case presentation, and when the patient agrees to the treatment, the dentist just can't stop talking. They go on and on about the interworking of the bonding procedure and details of the preparation design. The patient then becomes confused and scared, and fails to show up to their appointment.

The most important thing to remember when presenting your comprehensive treatment plan is when your patient says yes—STOP TALKING. This is your sign to change the subject, move on, and start talking about something they are interested in that doesn't include their teeth. You have accomplished a successful, effective case presentation when your patient says, *"Okay, I'll do it."* Use this opportunity to build even further rapport or just make the transfer to the team member who will schedule the appointment. The important thing to remember is to know when you have reached your goal, internally congratulate yourself, and move on.

Example:

Dentist: *Mrs. Tyler, on your upper left first molar you have a crown. Can you tell me when that crown was placed?*

Patient: *I'm not sure, but I think it was about eight or nine years ago.*

DR. MICHAEL DOLBY

Dentist:	*I see. In order for a crown to be effective, it must be sealed to your tooth. Sometimes, over time, bacteria or cavities can form on the root surface and get under your crown. Once the cavity has done this, the only solution is to remove the crown, so we can accurately remove the entire cavity and create a solid foundation for your tooth. Once that is completed, we will have our lab make a new all porcelain crown that more accurately fits and seals your tooth. I'm so happy you're not having any discomfort at this time. However, if this is not taken care of soon, the cavity may contact the nerve of the tooth, and then your tooth would require a root canal AND a new crown. I'm sure you would rather just have the new crown and avoid the whole root canal thing.*
Patient:	*Absolutely. I will make an appointment right away.*
Dentist:	*Great, I'll look forward to seeing you soon. By the way, how is your son, Alex, doing in college?*

Keep it simple and straightforward.

INTRA-ORAL PICTURES

The intra-oral camera is the most valuable piece of technical equipment in any dental office. This simple camera system allows your patients to see exactly what you're seeing. When used properly, it is responsible for creating the VALUE for the treatment you present to your patients.

Approximately 65 percent of all people are considered to be visual people. This means the vast majority of people tend to learn and absorb information by seeing it. You may have witnessed that some people will close their eyes to hear what someone is telling them. In fact, the next time you give someone directions, watch to see if they close their eyes in an attempt to visualize the route in their head.

The biggest challenge we face in dentistry is to build value for something that is out of sight out of mind and, in most instances, without discomfort. Since the majority of people need to see what you are talking about, it only makes sense to show them. Using intra-oral pictures is the key ingredient to significantly reducing this challenge. We have all heard the saying, *"A picture is worth a thousand words,"* and it is not uncommon for a patient to look at these pictures and, before you even comment, say, *"That doesn't look very good."* All you have to do now is go through the four stages of effective case presentation, and they will respond with *"How soon can you get me in?"*

It's no secret that the highest value for your treatment plan is created when your patient is actually present in your office. It's also no secret that this value has a tendency to decrease a soon as they walk out the door. You never know who the decision-maker in the home truly is, so one strategy to help reduce the "sticker shock" to their significant other is to send your patient home with printed pictures of the proposed treatment. Intra-oral pictures can help preserve that value you worked so hard to achieve. Pictures in hand that show why the treatment is needed are far more effective than just a fee slip showing how much the treatment will cost, which can be the difference in having your patient keep their scheduled appointment or not.

Your office policy should be that all patients are required to have a minimum of four intra-oral pictures taken during their hygiene appointments. Take a picture before you begin cleaning the lower anterior teeth, showing the accumulation of tartar that we all seem to develop. This is a powerful image that can't be missed. Then take two pictures of treatment areas that have been previously diagnosed, completed, or newly developed. Very often a previously completed treatment is out of site and out of mind, so for patients this can be a great opportunity to reinforce the high-quality work they have already receive in your office. For example, you can show how healthy the gum tissue is around a new porcelain crown and compare it to the inflammation and open margin around a crown you are proposing to replace.

At the end of the hygiene appointment, take a final picture of the lower anterior teeth with all the tartar removed. This dramatic before-and-after picture creates tons of value. Display all four pictures on the computer screen for the hygienist to reference during the hygiene appointment and for the doctor to review during the exam while the hygienist is "closing the loop."

When value has been created and your patient shows up for their restorative appointment, intra-oral pictures can continue to create even more value. During most of the dentistry we perform, our patients are not in any pain and can't see the teeth we are working on, so we have an opportunity to use our intra-oral photos to bring them into the process. Our assistants are taught to take a minimum of three pictures during restorative procedures. We take a "pre-prep" picture of the tooth, usually showing the broken-down silver filling or crown with an open margin that is going to be replaced. Next we take a "prep" picture with all the old restorative material removed, still showing the black grunge and decay that was living beneath the old restoration. We then take a "final" picture, showing the completed restoration.

All three of these pictures are ready for your patient to review at the end of the appointment. This provides them with something visual to reference. If they can see it, they can value it!

These restorative pre, prep, and post pictures are also valuable if a tooth remains sensitive after treatment. You are in a much better position when you can refer to a picture to remind your patient of the large cavity that was developing under their old crown or filling. Patients are quick to forget and more likely to understand just how compromised their tooth was before treatment when they have a picture to refer to.

We also include these pictures with the submission of our insurance claims. This allows the insurance examiners to understand the case in a more intimate level. Combining pictures with your narrative description can mean the difference between an easy approval or having the insurance company ask for additional information.

There is no question intra-oral pictures increase the value of the services you provide. The more value you create, the more likely it will be that the patient shares their experience with their family and friends, and, more importantly, refers new patients to your practice.

PHASING TREATMENT PLANS

You can be certain that most of the time your patient will be slightly to moderately overwhelmed with any amount of treatment you are proposing, so it's important to acknowledge this. When treatment plans involve more than a few teeth, it can be beneficial to direct your patient's focus on the area of most concern. Present everything you found that needs attention, but avoid overwhelming the patient with too much detail. For example, if the patient needs three crowns, there is no need to explain each tooth in detail because really describing one will allow your patient to understand the reason for all the others. Choosing a priority area, especially for new patients that have never had a treatment experience with you, can be wise. Most patients have some level of apprehension, and past experiences play a huge role in a patient's decision to move forward with any treatment until they know that everything is going to be okay and you not going to hurt them. Once they have experienced a stress-free appointment with you, they are likely to move rapidly through the remainder of their treatment plan.

Your goal is to diagnose everything that needs to be corrected and present the highest priority areas. Build value for that treatment and then let the patient decide how they would like to proceed. I've had patients with a quadrant of crowns and fillings to correct, that insisted on completing one tooth at a time. I will always honor my patient's wishes, but I have found that once they are in your chair and you have completed the "one tooth" with no discomfort as they requested, they are likely to allow you to continue with the remainder of the treatment at the next appointment.

Phasing treatment plans is an important strategy, especially with new patients. This strategy goes a long way towards getting patients to begin treatment, which gives you an opportunity to create value for the rest of the treatment plan.

MAXIMIZE YOUR TREATMENT OPPORTUNITIES

Master Confrontational Tolerance

Build Rapport

Ask Permission

Comprehensive Diagnosis

Effective Case Presentation

Utilize Intra-Oral Photos

DR. MICHAEL DOLBY

FINANCIAL AGREEMENTS

Collections

Have you ever gone to the grocery store or to your favorite coffee house, and when it came time to pay for your items, you told the cashier, *"Just send me a bill"*? These people would look at you with a blank stare as to what in the world you were talking about. However, the health care industry is really hesitant when it comes to asking for payment for the services they have rendered.

The *"Just bill me"* mentality arose from the introduction of insurance. In the early years of dental insurance, most patients and doctors knew the insurance reimbursement would cover the doctor's fee, so it seemed redundant to ask the patient to pay for something the insurance company was going to pay for anyway. Today, we all know this is a far different story. Insurance reimbursements are covering less and less, and, more importantly, the time it takes to actually receive your reimbursement is taking longer and longer. Health care practices are finding it more difficult to manage the finances of their practices when it takes 30–45 days to receive any payment for their services.

Student loans, practice overhead, and team salaries don't get paid with IOUs, so it's essential that your practice remains profitable. If the team member you assigned to address financial arrangements is intimidated or hesitant when discussing this sensitive subject, it's critical to the existence of your office to find someone who can handle this extremely important job.

I have seen doctors pressuring their team to get patients into the schedule, and in response to this pressure, team members encourage patients to schedule their appointments, assuring them that everything will be covered through their dental insurance. Most patients will usually agree to this arrangement because, in their minds, it's basically free, and the schedule gets full. However, there are only two outcomes when you avoid making financial arrangements with your patients before starting treatment: (1) You will lose them now, or (2) you will lose them later! The relationship with your patient will certainly be damaged when you eventually have to inform them their insurance only covered half of their new bridge.

Nobody likes to be surprised, especially when it comes to money, so making solid financial arrangements with every patient is an absolute must for your practice to be successful. This, however, does NOT mean that your office becomes a bank that carries balances or makes in-house loans. Today there are too many third party lending companies, such as Care Credit, that are in the business of making these types of loans. In fact, do you really want to extend a loan to a patient that Care Credit deemed not credit-worthy? We are in the business of dentistry, so let the banking professionals do what they do and leave the credit lending practice to someone else.

A strategy I have seen too many rely on is simply sending patients to collections if they cannot recover their money. This is definitely NOT a strategy you should ever rely on. When a patient defaults on a dental bill, it's usually because of a poor job of handling financial arrangements in the first place. When this happens, you need to take full responsibility and learn from the experience, and, in many cases, you may even have to suffer the loss. The negative image created by sending your patient to collections is not worth the slim chance that you will ever recover any of the money anyway. You can count on this person sharing with everyone that you are just a greedy dentist. You decide how you want to be known in your community. After all, this started with a simple lack of financial arrangements before treatment was started.

Once it becomes clear that your patient is going to default on their outstanding balance, you are better off sending them a handwritten note saying that you understand they must be going through some tough financial times. Tell them that you are putting their account on hold, and whenever they can pay will be great with you. This will blow your patient's mind because if they owe you money, trust me, they owe a bunch of other people also. You can be certain they are receiving nothing but collection notices, so when this comes in the mail, they will be overjoyed. You might as well keep your rapport because getting mad and taking action won't get you paid any sooner. However, this act of kindness will be shared with everyone they meet, so your brand will continue to grow strong. And you never know, your bill might even move to the top of their "to-pay" list.

It's important to always remember that people will buy anything they value. If you have done an outstanding job with your case presentation, creating value for the proposed treatment, then your patients will find a way to financially afford to have their dentistry completed. It's really that simple. Sometimes our emotions can take over, and we want our patients to accept our treatment plans so bad that we find creative ways to get them in the schedule, even if it means compromising financial arrangements. The amazing thing about a patient's pending dental treatment is that it never goes away; the treatment just changes. The crown you diagnosed last year will usually turn into a root canal along with a new crown. It's just a matter of time. So don't compromise the financial health of your practice if your patients decide to hold off on their treatment.

My uncle once gave me some great advice. He told me, *"You don't have to do all the dentistry in one day."* If you master confrontational tolerance, diagnose comprehensively, present with absolute certainty, and make solid financial arrangements, then your patients will make the right choices.

MASTERING INSURANCE

GOING TO WAR

Dental insurance seems to be the most common frustration among just about every dental practice I have come across. The increasing amount of time and documentation that is being required for the simplest of procedures is forcing many offices to hire a fulltime person just to keep up. Not to mention the follow-up that now seems mandatory with just about every claim if you want to actually get paid.

You would think the dental insurance companies would cater to their member dentists and make the process as easy and seamless as possible. However, after 20 years in private practice, one thing is very clear: Dental insurance companies are in business to make money, and every decision they make is based on that principle. I don't care if their motto is *"Started by dentists, for dentists,"* like Delta Dental, profit is their main goal, so you can expect to have every claim and every diagnosis you submit challenged.

For just a minute, try to imagine just how much money the insurance companies might make from just the interest, simply by delaying payment of your claim 30, 60, or 90 days. Trust me, that number is huge, resulting in a strong motivation to have your claims delayed or denied. When you think about this, it's a great strategy for the insurance company because they aren't upsetting their customer, the policyholder, because most payments are sent directly to the dental office, so they are really just inconveniencing the dentist. We can complain all we want and say it's not fair, but, trust me, it won't get our claims reimbursed any more quickly. However, what we can do is learn to play the game better than anyone else.

I have to say the team members who deal with this endless stream of dental insurance claims, necessary follow-ups, and requests for additional information deserve a medal, an award, or some sort of special recognition. This is one of the toughest, most frustrating duties in the office. Hours can be spent on the phone trying to resolve even the simplest request, only to end up getting put on hold and doing it all over again. Creating systems to support this task is essential for the long-term success of your practice.

GETTING ORGANIZED

Being extremely organized is the first step in your fight to minimize the frustrations that come with submitting claims. Dental insurance companies are too busy to challenge every submission, so they focus on the claims that are an easy target to send through the lengthy review process. For example, claims that have weak narratives, the wrong coding, or procedures that aren't even covered by the plan are easily rejected. To beat them at their own game, you must first have a general understanding of your patients' insurance plans and what is required to be included with each claim. If a patient's insurance plan requires an x-ray of the apex for all crowns that have had previous root canal therapy and you send in a bite-wing x-ray, you can expect the claim to be rejected. Also, if you submit a claim for an onlay and in the narrative you fail to mention which cusp was under-supported or describe why an indirect restoration would not work, that claim is coming back too.

To beat them at their own game, you must eliminate any reason they can think of to reject your claim. The more information you can include, the better. Provide every claim with detailed narratives about the procedure that describes when and why the treatment was chosen for a particular patient. Send x-rays, study models, and even impressions if necessary. You want the evaluator who is assigned to your claim to be inundated with information and justification for that treatment, so they will quickly approve your claim for payment.

An effective strategy is to send pre-op, mid-prep, and post-prep intra-oral photos. A pre-prep picture will show the defective restoration before you have started treatment. The mid-prep picture is taken when you have removed the existing filling material, exposing the decay that lies underneath. Finally, the post-prep picture will show the finished restoration or the prepared tooth foundation that will be going to the lab for an indirect restoration These pictures will allow the examiner to completely understand what you were faced with prior to any treatment and the decision process that led you to choose this particular restoration.

Think about this from the insurance examiner's point of view. They are asked to make a decision on your claim, and all you sent them was a cone-cut x-ray and a one-sentence narrative. The examiners might seem unreasonable most of the time, but they certainly are not mind readers. The more information you can provide, the easier it is for them to completely understand your restorative choices, thus allowing them to make a more informed decision about your claim, usually with a positive result.

All insurance claims submitted the same day!

It's no secret the front office can be a very busy place, with patients checking in and out, phones ringing, questions about financial arrangements, scheduling appointments, etc. When the proper business systems have not been created for handling the abundance of insurance claims, the front office can quickly find itself overwhelmed. When that happens, the processing of your insurance claims can sometimes be put off until the next day. However, when the next day arrives, the busyness of the practice returns, and the claims go, once again, unprocessed. I have evaluated offices where stacks of insurance claims were sitting in a file drawer having never been submitted for payment. Can you imagine performing all of that dentistry essentially for FREE? Unfortunately, this happens far too often, and, to make matters worse, dentists are usually completely unaware this is going on.

Every insurance claim created during the workday must be processed and submitted with all the appropriate documentation before the end of the same day. This system is critical and can mean the difference between success and failure for the practice. When the habit is created of putting off the daily processing of insurance claims, not only will the practice suffer financially, but patients will also start to lose faith because of your lack of organization and handling of their claims. Your job is to make sure patients' dental claims are paid quickly, so the practice can recover the expenses that went into making the claims. If a refund is in order, your patient should receive that reimbursement promptly. When this process takes too long because of disorganization, your patient will think you are holding onto their money, and nothing ruins a relationship faster than a dispute over the almighty dollar. Having a system that keeps you organized in this department will preserve the value for our services that we are always trying to create.

DR. MICHAEL DOLBY

Outstanding Insurance Claims

Your practice management software can be an invaluable tool when it comes to handling your insurance claims. Once a week, it is crucial to run the report for the *outstanding insurance claims*. This report lists all the claims that have been sent to the insurance company and the dates they were sent. When you make this report part of your weekly routine, it will show you exactly how long claims have been pending payment and provides you the opportunity to follow up with the insurance company as to what might be causing the delay. Often a claim sits on an insurance examiner's desk because they need an answer to a simple question and haven't found the time to call you. When you take this pro-active initiative, you will find the payment process will be much quicker. Those who sit and wait, unfortunately, get served last!

Procedures Not Attached to Claims

You might be amazed at how many procedures are floating around in your practice management software that have not been attached to the patient's chart or submitted with any insurance claim. Another very important report in your weekly insurance management system is to review the procedures that are not attached to any insurance claims. As I stated before, procedures end up on this list when treatment was posted into the computer but failed to be attached to the insurance claim.

When you have treated several teeth in one appointment, it can be easy to forget to include one tooth, and these so-called "little" procedures can add up quickly. A weekly review of this report will allow you to properly account for all treatment that has been completed in the practice.

Insurance Claims to Process

We have already stressed the importance of submitting all of your claims at the end of the day. A quick glance at the Insurance Claims to Process report will ensure that all claims have been accounted for, submitted, and are on their way to being paid. This list should be a clean slate at the end of each day.

Along with the review of your Outstanding Claims report, the Insurance Aging report will show how long you have been waiting for claims to be processed and paid. It's common for a team member to follow the correct steps in processing a claim on the same day as the treatment and then simply forget about it. It would be great if the insurance companies treated you like an actual customer and made an effort to process the claim promptly, alerting you when they need more information without submitting an entire new claim—but that is not the case.

The Insurance Aging report gives you the opportunity to follow up with the insurance company and get answers as to why the claim is taking so long to process. Remember what I said in the beginning of this chapter: The insurance company has really no incentive to process your claim promptly because they can profit from the interest their money is generating by just letting it sit in the bank. So it's up to you to manage every one of your claims and know where they are in the process of payment at all times.

CHALLENGE THE INSURANCE COMPANIES

Dental insurance companies have become so big that it can be intimidating to think you have a chance in challenging any of their decisions. They seem to have influence over your clinical decisions, whether or not you can ask your patients for payment, and they certainly have influence over your fees. But you do have a voice, and, more importantly, you have the right to defend the way you choose to practice. If enough of us do this, individuals and employers might start considering that traditional dental insurance is not the best choice for themselves or their employees, and look for other options, such as medical health savings accounts or being self-insured.

The dental community must stand together and challenge the insurance companies when they obviously do not have our patients' best interests in mind. Be that voice for yourself, your dental community, and your patients! We have the power together to limit the influence these companies have on the way we choose to practice dentistry. Unlike our medical colleagues that allowed the insurance companies to literally take complete control over their profession, let us all commit to never stop the fight!

DR. MICHAEL DOLBY

MARKETING

You are what you repeatedly do.
Excellence is not an event. It is a habit.
—Aristotle

When we think of marketing, we usually think of magazine ads, billboards, TV, etc. By definition, marketing is the process of informing your customers the value of your products and services. However, marketing is really a part of everything we do in our practice, and, as you can imagine, this is a critical business function for not only attracting new patients, but for the continued growth of your practice.

For the longest time, dentists considered marketing their dental practices to be degrading, not only to themselves but also to the entire profession. Many believed that if you had to advertise for people to come see you, then you must not be a very good dentist! Fortunately, times have changed and so have the opinions regarding the promotion of your practice. Most state dental boards have detailed guidelines on what type of advertising is acceptable, but the general consensus is that advertising is fine as long as it's done in a professional manner.

I am a huge supporter of marketing your practice professionally while not devaluing or degrading the profession in any way. However, when dentists direct their marketing efforts towards half-priced crowns and free cleanings, this accomplishes only one thing—it positions price as the highest value. In return, you are going to attract people that value price over the quality of their care, your team, customer service, etc., and, as soon as the "free" stuff is gone, so are they. Don't get me wrong, I want to save money just like the next guy, but I believe that most people are not willing to save money if it means compromising the actual dental care they receive.

Marketing your services and special training to attract great, long-term patients that will refer their family and friends will always serve your practice better. When I mentioned earlier about the true value of a patient, I made reference to the small amount of value a patient has that only comes into your office when they are in pain or so infrequently that you wonder if they are actually still a patient versus the value of a patient that refers consistently their family and friends to your practice, even if they don't have any dentistry to do themselves.

Remember, busy doesn't equal profitable, and it certainly doesn't mean you're growing your practice. If your marketing efforts are price and free stuff driven, you can be assured that you will be busy running from chair to chair, taking very little to the bank, and wondering why your practice is not growing.

Modern marketing concepts acknowledge that everything matters in marketing, and that a broad and integrated perspective is necessary for developing, designing, and implementing a successful marketing program. There are four main components to a successful marketing program that you must consider:

Relationship Marketing

Internal Marketing

External-Brand Marketing

Socially Responsible Marketing

Relationship Marketing:

This type of marketing places the emphasis on the value of the relationship between your team and the patients you serve. The goal is to provide outstanding customer service, create rapport, and build value for your services, and to create a strong foundation for the relationship. People buy from people or businesses they like. It's just that simple. We have discussed the importance of creating value and developing great rapport with every patient, and that is the essence of relationship marketing.

Often we think the relationship marketing only happens while we are in the office and caring for patients. However, this also holds true outside of the office. How your team members conduct themselves in public or outside of the office has a direct reflection on the practice. When you see one of your patients out in public, do you go out of your way to say hello or do you pretend you don't know that person? When you meet a person outside of the office that is new to the area, do you give them your business card and invite them to your office for a complimentary exam, or do you avoid the subject? These marketing strategies are necessary for every team member to adopt and should be an integral part of the practice culture.

All team members should have individual business cards with an incentive, such as a complimentary exam or discounted bleach trays. Whether they are attending a chamber of commerce event, participating in a leads group or any other social community event, these are all marketing opportunities for your team members to invite new patients to the practice.

Relationship marketing is an important aspect of your marketing efforts and includes the active involvement of your entire team.

Internal Marketing

This is sometimes called *inward facing* marketing, where the focus is on your existing patients who are already invested in your practice. It is the most important area of marketing for you and your team to focus on and works in direct correlation with relationship marketing. Internal marketing is where the most successful dental practices spend 80 percent of their marketing budget. Why? Because they know there is not a better audience to create a stream of new patients to the practice than your existing clientele. Think about it, your current patients already know you and your team, they know the quality of dentistry you provide and your level of customer service, they know your location and hours, so naturally they would be your best marketing advocates. However, when offices are not seeing the amount of referrals they would like, they may indeed be the very thing stopping patients from consistently referring their friends and family to the practice.

Your patients must be given direction and permission to invite others to join your practice. We have all heard patients ask us: *"Are you accepting new patients?"* I think we all just assume that patients know we are ALWAYS taking new patients, but the reality is they don't. This thought process happens because many of our physician colleagues are indeed not accepting new patients, along with the fact dentists and their teams simply do not consistently ask their existing patients to refer new clients to them. So if patients are unaware we are accepting new patients and we don't ask, then how can we expect this to happen?

I have found the most effective strategy to consistently get your current patients to refer friends and family to your practice is by establishing a "Care to Share" referral program. This program is easy to implement and provides a credit for any new patient referred to the practice, along with the new patient receiving a credit they can apply towards their first appointment.

I do realize it can feel awkward and uncomfortable to just ask a patient out of the blue for their referral, making you feel like a used car salesman. However, I have found that the best time to introduce the subject of referrals into the conversation is right after a patient gives you a compliment. We have all experienced when a patient will take a moment and compliment us on our professionalism, the quality of our work, or a particular team member, and that is the perfect time to follow that compliment with an explanation of the Care to Share referral program. Let your patient know how much you enjoy having them in your practice and even emphasize that in a perfect world you wish all of the patients in your practice could be just like them. Your patient will love the compliment, and they most likely will refer another great patient to your practice. Hand them a Care to Share card and explain that for every new patient they refer to your office, they will receive a $25 credit on their account, and their referral will also receive a $25 credit. You can certainly create any incentive you want, but the point is that you are not only giving them permission to refer new patients to your office, but also providing them a small incentive to do so.

The tangible Care to Share card is an important ingredient to this system because it reinforces or reminds your patient to refer friends and family long after the conversation in your office is over. Since they have something tangible to give a potential new patient, they are likely to keep this card close by.

Now you will have a system in place that has the potential to be the key ingredient to increasing new patients to your practice. However, it's critical that everyone on your team participates, giving every patient the permission to start referring.

External Brand Marketing

When a practice is experiencing decreased production and, more importantly, collections, the knee-jerk response is *"We need more new patients!"* Without a marketing plan or strategy in place, thousands of dollars can be spent on direct mail ads, billboards, television, newsletters, etc. without much return on the investment. Don't get me wrong, external marketing efforts are necessary and can be productive, but in the dental profession, it can feel more like fishing for patients. You throw your marketing piece out there in the sea of advertisers, and you're not really sure what you'll catch or what type of patients will arrive in your office.

External brand marketing is the development of a consistent message across a myriad of marketing channels that must be congruent with the high-quality patients you are trying to attract. In this context, "branding" refers to the philosophy and culture of your practice. What do you want to be known for in your community? Are you a children's practice? A cosmetically focused practice? A laser practice? A CAD-CAM practice? Whatever you enjoy doing and want to be known for, you must focus on getting that message out to your community and potential new patients. Remember, the worst thing you can do is try and be everything to everybody because you will soon find that you end up being nothing to nobody!

I've seen dentists change their advertising every month, promoting themselves as something different each time. I expect this is the result of the latest continuing education course where the presenter convinced them the latest niche is all that it will take to get them to the top. This strategy will only confuse your potential patient base, and when patients are confused about who you are, they will be hesitant to establish themselves with your practice.

Creating a brand is essential to the growth and prosperity of your practice, so think long and hard about what you want to be known for in your market and what you can do to support that image. Consistency with your brand message will lead to congruency within your practice, and that, in turn, will leave no doubt in your potential patients' minds of exactly who you are and how they can benefit from your services.

Socially Responsible Marketing

Social responsibility in marketing is often discussed along with the topic of ethics. It refers to marketing activities that are not harmful to your colleagues or the dental profession as a whole, with either the products you are offering or service claims you are promoting.

A Colorado dentist once advertised that he could cure multiple sclerosis if you had him remove all of your silver fillings. As you would expect, this dentist lost his license and is serving jail time over these claims and practices. I realize this is an extreme example, but dentists should avoid advertising treatments they cannot duplicate with every patient. For example, advertising that you are *"pain-free"* or that you can make a patient look like their favorite movie star is irresponsible and frankly untrue. We all know that changing a person's smile will definitely make them look better. However, you're only changing their teeth, not their body, height, weight, etc. You will make them look better and possibly more attractive, but they will still have the weathered skin, droopy eyelids, and saggy chin! You get the point. As far as pain-free goes, I'm sure 99% of your patients feel little, if no, discomfort, but we all have that special group of patients that feels everything. So making these claims will often give you more trouble than it's worth.

Instead, promote what you can offer patients regarding quality of care, outstanding customer service, and a caring environment. If you stay within the guidelines of your local dental board's marketing practices and only make claims that you would make to a friend or family member, then you will be promoting your practice with socially responsible marketing strategies. Make a commitment to practice and market with integrity, and your reputation with be held at the highest level.

A MILLION DOLLAR PRACTICE WITH ONLY 1,000 PATIENTS

Many dentists believe they need thousands of patients to have a successful practice. The truth is, it's not how many patients you have, but how efficient and productive you are with current patients. I have consulted practices that had more than 5,000 patient charts but were still failing financially. How could any practice with that many patients have holes in their schedule?

The fact is, without the correct business systems efficiently guiding a patient through your practice, the number of patient charts could be 100,000, and it wouldn't change a thing. To reach $1 million in production can be accomplished with far fewer patients than you might think.

Let's discuss the example of creating a million dollar practice with just 1,000 patients. If each of those 1,000 patients needs the basics of two hygiene visits per year at a nominal fee of $70, two exams at $45, and four bitewing x-rays at $50, the total would be $280,000. If you include one periodontal procedure on only half of those patients, with an average fee of $200, and one major procedure on just 70 percent of the patients, at an average fee of $900, the total would be $730,000. Combine that with the $280,000 from the hygiene services, and you have a grand total of $1,010,000.

I think you will agree this is certainly not an exaggerated example. Consider that we haven't even accounted for cosmetic procedures, laser therapy, night guard appliances, orthodontics, endodontics, implants, and oral surgery, just to name a few. Imagine including a few of these procedures, and there is no telling what kind of number you could reach.

The fact is, the average dental practice produces $500,000 to $650,000 per year with 1,500 to 1,800 patients. Kind of a shame based on the example I just gave, don't you think? Obviously, these practices have not mastered clinical efficiency, along with other critical business systems, or they would easily have hit the million-dollar mark. It doesn't take an overabundance of patients to make your practice grow, yet still the most common request among struggling offices is how to get more new patients. While obtaining new patients is an important function of growing your practice, it's clearly not the barrier that keeps most practices from achieving success.

My point is this: With an efficient, well-managed practice, creating a million dollars in production is not only realistic—it's achievable.

A Million Dollar Practice with only 1,000 Patients!

2 hygiene visits per year at an average of $70 each = $140,000

2 exams per year at an average of $45 each = $90,000

4 bitewing x-rays at an average of $50 = $50,000

1 major procedure on just 70% of patient base at an average of $900 = $630,000

1 perio procedure on just 50% of patient base at an average of $200 = $100,000

TOTAL: $1,010,000

CONTROLLING THE OVERHEAD MONSTER

Are you as profitable as you should be?

*The key to success is for you to make a habit throughout your life
of doing the things you fear.*
—Brian Tracy

Dentists sometimes have a unique way of showing their superiority over their colleagues. We can see this as far back as the early 1900s when Painless Parker measured his success by the number of teeth he strung around his neck at the end of the day!

Boasting of high production numbers seems to be the new benchmark of success for dentists. The quest for larger production numbers has prompted many dentists to prematurely expand their offices to accommodate more chairs, build multiple offices, or even add associate doctors. The use of production numbers as a measure of financial success is stretching the truth.

Managing a busy office and your team, staying current with the latest dental techniques, and keeping patients happy can take dentists to the breaking point once they discover their so-called high-producing dental practice is experiencing financial challenges because of out-of-control overhead.

I often hear doctors say what they really want is to just "do the dentistry," and not have to figure out the "numbers" part of the practice or be the leader their team wants. It would be great if our practices could afford the luxury of a chief financial officer, but for most of us, this is not an option. A clear understanding of your financial position is an absolute must if you are to experience the maximum returns you have worked so hard to achieve.

KNOWING YOUR NUMBERS

The great economist Peter Drucker said, *"You can only manage what you measure."* Unfortunately, many doctors rarely know the true financial health of their own practices. When asked how many new patients they saw the previous month, I usually hear them say something like, "*Well, I think about average.*" When asked what their gross production was, they often reply, "*About the same as the previous month.*" With responses like this, it's no wonder the majority of dental offices are not as profitable as they should be. The financial numbers of your practice are like the speedometer in a car. They tell you if your practice is growing or shrinking, profitable or in the red, and they need to be accurate.

Before the 1990s, it was rare to hear about a dental practice closing its doors because it was essentially bankrupt. Today that news is all too common. In the so-called Golden Age of Dentistry, a practice could survive with an inflated, or what I call "fat," overhead and still make a good living. These practices may not have been as profitable as they could have, but at the end of the month, everybody seemed to have their needs met, so there was little motivation to squeeze the fat out of the practice. In today's competitive market and tough economy, these types of sloppy business practices will not allow dentists to have their needs met, or, for that matter, even survive.

Dentists must focus on the financial health of their practices. Accurate financial monitors can be an essential tool in detecting trouble before it becomes too cumbersome to correct.

THE BIG THREE

Controlling overhead and the financial health of your practice is not as difficult as it may appear. If you can learn to prepare a crown, then you can certainly learn what it takes to keep your practice profitable. There are a few critical areas to manage that have a massive impact on your financial future. I call them *"The BIG THREE."*

These three categories play an important role in the successful overhead management of your practice and account for approximately 50% of your total practice overhead. If you can commit yourself to mastering control over The BIG THREE, then you will reap the financial rewards for the rest of your career.

THE BIG THREE

Team Compensation

Dental Supplies

Laboratory Expenses

By converting "The BIG THREE" categories into individual percentages, you can easily manage your overhead. I want to be very clear that ALL overhead percentage calculations are based on NET COLLECTIONS, not production. A simple way to remember this is that you can only spend what you deposit in the bank. With this in mind, take the total expense in each of these categories and divide them into the total net collection number for the month or year-to-date (YTD). For example, at year-end, if your total team compensation is $110,000 and your total net collections are $500,000, you simply divide these numbers to determine your total team overhead percentage. For this example it would be 22 percent.

TEAM COMPENSATION

Unfortunately, the first place most doctors look to "cut overhead" is by trimming the number of team members they employ or, worse, reducing their compensation. There is no quicker way to suck the energy out of a practice than to reduce someone's pay. Sometimes reducing the size of your team is a viable strategy, but for the majority of practices, this is not the case.

Practices that are experiencing high team compensation overhead are usually not overstaffed; they are simply underproducing with the team they have in place. If you have one hygienist, one front office receptionist, and one dental assistant and you are still having challenges getting your staff overhead percentage under control, then cutting the size of your team is certainly NOT the answer.

The most efficient strategy to control this overhead category without reducing staff is to simply increase your production and net collections. Your total team compensation is a relatively fixed number, so when collections reach a certain point, the impact of your team compensation percentage, in regard to overhead, will be reduced. Maximizing the efficiency of your team is the primary goal when it comes to controlling your overhead.

Calculating your total team compensation is probably the most controversial area of overhead management regarding what is included in this category. I have heard every explanation and rationalization from "management experts" around the country about what should be included in or left out of this figure.

From my perspective, it's as simple as this: You include everything that it costs for every member on your team. You don't make it any more complicated. Include your team members' salaries or hourly wage compensations, any extra benefits, taxes, employee perks, etc.—everything that makes up their TOTAL compensation packages. Think of it this way: If it costs the practice money to have this team member show up at your office, then it should be included in the total.

An appropriate overhead percentage for the total team compensation should be between 18 and 25 percent of total yearly net collections. If you have trouble controlling this percentage, the most effective line of defense is to find ways to increase production and net collections with the smallest, most efficient team possible.

DENTAL SUPPLIES

In this advanced age of bonding, all-ceramic crowns, CAD-CAM technology, and other high-tech gadgets, it's easy for doctors to be drawn into buying all the latest materials and high-tech toys. They watch as their supply room shelves grow, crowded with high-tech promises that did not live up to expectations. The incredible arsenal of supplies that are required today for the most routine dental procedure is amazing. Part of mastering dental supply overhead is to master clinical efficiency with your clinical setup and to obtain the best materials at the best prices.

It's okay to try new products, and I certainly recommend that all doctors do this to stay current with the best that dentistry can offer. However, smart buying decisions are the key to managing your business. Don't be tempted to be "the first on the block" to use a particular new, "revolutionary" product. Use products that have solid names behind them, along with credible research and proven track records. The first generation of most products tends to be more of a market test. The reliable, proven products emerge in the second and third generations.

Negotiating prices with dental supply companies is a necessity for all practices. Once you have discovered the core supplies you need in your office, find a reliable company that will provide you with a discount if you make a commitment to buy all of your supplies through them. You will be surprised just how willing these companies are to offer you special incentives to earn your business. If you don't ask, you'll never know!

What I do not recommend is having a dental assistant spend hours on the Internet or buried in dental catalogs finding the "lowest prices" on supplies. Saving a few bucks on a Brand X bonding agent may end up costing you more because of remakes and losses in patient confidence.

You should strive for an overhead percentage in the dental supply category of between 6 and 8 percent of total yearly net collections. It's important to know that some months may be over your allotted percentage. However, your year-to-date percentage is the true indicator that you are keeping on track and managing this department appropriately.

LABORATORY EXPENSE

I've seen some doctors brag about paying high fees for a single restoration, as if it is "successful" to increase your overhead in this area of your practice. Some dentists will say, *"But you have to pay more to receive high-quality work."* I'm not suggesting that you send your work to East Asia for $39 crowns made of aluminum. I am suggesting that you closely examine what you are getting for your money like in any successful business. Ask yourself—Would it be possible to receive the same high level of quality at a reduced price from another company?

I have had the opportunity to speak with many of the different laboratory representatives producing high-quality dental restorations, and several indicated they would be willing to provide a significant discount if a practice made a commitment to use their lab exclusively. Just like the dental supply example, wouldn't any smart businessperson be willing to provide some sort of incentive in return for a constant influx of work? The answer is most definitely YES.

Lab expenses can also be an indicator for how comprehensive the practice is diagnosing. If a practice is experiencing problems with their gross production number, they most likely have fallen prey to confrontational tolerance. They slowly start diagnosing only what the patient will accept or what their insurance will pay for. Indirect restorations, such as crowns and onlays, begin to disappear from treatment plans while more direct placement four- and five-surface fillings start showing up. An acceptable percentage for your total laboratory expenses should be in the range of 10 to 12 percent, but this figure can be as low as 7 to 10 percent with an office that has efficiently incorporated CAD-CAM technology.

MARKETING EXPENSE

Marketing is not listed with the BIG THREE, but it is an expense that must be managed. Often practices spend thousands of dollars on expensive TV, radio, and print ads without properly researching to see if these avenues will attract the type of patient they are seeking. Your goal is to have your marketing expense in the range of 2 to 5 percent of your total overhead. A start-up practice, however, may see expenses in the 5 to 8 percent range, then taper back to a normal percentage as the practice becomes busier.

As we discussed before, the most successful practices spend approximately 80 percent of their marketing budgets on internal marketing. So don't get caught up in trying to go head-to-head with the external marketing efforts of *"Corporate Discount Dentistry."* Just because another dentist is being financially irresponsible with their marketing efforts doesn't mean you have to follow.

TAKE CONTROL—TODAY!

We discussed earlier that what you focus on, you receive. This could not be more important when it comes to controlling your overhead. By proactively managing *THE BIG THREE*—your team's total compensation, dental supplies, and laboratory expenses—you will find yourself more than on your way to a successful and profitable practice.

DR. MICHAEL DOLBY

The remaining overhead categories are essentially fixed expenses, and there is not much you can do proactively to control them. For example, your office rent will likely not change month-to-month, and the light bill is relatively consistent. However, the management of practice overhead is an annual, quarterly, monthly, and even daily event.

If you are to achieve the goal of *Controlling the Overhead Monster*, you must be willing to step up and tame this beast. You can only manage what you measure, so rely on your Practice Success Monitors (explained in the next chapter) to accurately show areas where you can improve. Don't get caught up in the bragging of big production numbers that you read about in dental journals or hear at dental meetings. What you take home matters, not what you produce. Let those guys work twice as hard for half the money. You know with certainty that maximizing your production combined with the lowest overhead is the true definition of financial success in the dental office.

Overhead Percentages

	Poor	Good	Outstanding
Team Compensation	27%	23%	19%
Dental Supplies	10%	8%	6%
Laboratory Expense	12%	10%	10%
Marketing	5%	3%	3%
Office	7%	5%	5%
Continuing Education	4%	3%	2%
Administrative	6%	5%	4%
Miscellaneous	8%	6%	6%
Total Overhead	**79%**	**63%**	**55%**
Net Profit	**21%**	**37%**	**45%**

PRACTICE SUCCESS MONITORS

As we discussed earlier, Peter Drucker tells us that you can't effectively manage what you don't track; therefore, we must review certain departments within our practice on a regular basis to gain a clear picture of how the practice is performing. Waiting until the end of the year to examine your profit and loss, and to balance sheet statements, which most of us don't understand anyway, provides no opportunity for you to make any corrections to get your practice back on course and moving towards your goals.

The month-end reports that you often get from your practice management software definitely have their pros and cons; however, they can provide you with valuable tracking reports to assist you in managing your practice. The challenge is that it usually takes multiple steps to get that information, and what we really want is to see everything together in one place and scaled down to the most basic level. A single-page Practice Success Monitor would allow a quick assessment on how the practice is doing regarding the most important categories of the practice. It would show numbers for the current month and compare the year-to-date numbers, all at a glance. I believe the biggest reason most dentists don't consistently review the finances of their practice is because these numbers are not that easy to obtain or to understand.

At Triumph Dental we have created a one-page "Practice Success Monitor" that is easy to understand and shows everything you need to proactively manage your practice, all on one page. At a glance, you can easily see each department and track your percentages towards your goals. You can use this monitor to review with your team and your coach each month to assure your practice is operating at peak level.

When reviewing the Practice Success Monitor, we obviously want to know our **gross production**, as it relates to the goal we have set for the practice. This number is simply all the treatment services the practice produced that month. It should be broken down further to evaluate your gross production per day and per hour to show you exactly how efficiently your practice is performing. Reviewing this number will remind you of the value of your time, which you can easily forget. Just because you have been practicing for 10 or more years and you can repair a mesial/ distal fracture on tooth #9 in your sleep, does not mean that you should give those production dollars away. I'm all for giving away a certain amount of production for charity, but when you know what you are worth per day and per hour, you might want to think twice about giving this away so indiscriminately.

It is also important to know exactly what makes up the gross-production number. This allows you to evaluate how efficiently the two producing departments, doctor and hygiene, are contributing to the total production number. The Practice Success Monitor has a category set up for each doctor and hygienist, showing his or her individual production goal along with his or her actual production for the month. This total is broken down further to determine the production per patient visit.

An acceptable range you should be shooting for would be between $600 and $800 per patient visit for the doctor, and $180 and $225 for the hygiene department. This allows you to clearly see the true value of each patient in your schedule. If a patient is a no-show or cancels on short notice, this lost production opportunity can add up quickly and negatively affect the success of your practice. Strive for your hygiene department to contribute at least 25 percent of the practice's total gross production while the doctor's production makes up the remaining percentage. This is an indicator that will let you know if your hygiene department is performing at an optimum level.

It should be no surprise that **total collections** are extremely important. This is how your practice continues to stay alive and pay its bills. However, it can be an eye-opening experience to see just how much you are collecting compared to what you have achieved in gross production.

When you track this number, it can be humbling to discover the actual amount you are writing off. Those amazing PPO and managed-care dental insurance plans you signed up for, not to mention what your patients still owe you, affect your bottom line. It is essential to the success of your practice that you know the ratio of your collections, as compared to gross production, along with where these funds are coming from.

We can track these figures on the Practice Success Monitor in three specific areas: (1) the percentage of total collections as it relates to gross production; (2) the percentage of total collections from over-the-counter payments; and (3) the breakdown of accounts receivables. These three categories accurately account for all the revenue your practice has produced. When you know where the money is, you have a much better chance of having that money end up in your bank account.

When your practice collects at least 50 percent of its total production at the time of service, you are creating value for the dentistry your patient has just received. I think we have all experienced when we get things for free or pay for them later, the value of those services seems to diminish. For me, it has never made sense to "bill" everything to the insurance company and wait to see what they will cover before your patient settles their end of the treatment cost. With a little research of your patients' dental insurance plans, you should be able to estimate their financial portion and create a culture where patients are expected to pay at least this portion at the time of service. You cannot afford to wait 30 to 60 days for the insurance company to reimburse you, then send your patient a statement, and wait another 15 to 30 days for that payment.

Your overall total collection goal should be between 95 and 98 percent of your total net collectable production. The **net collection** number is generated by your total gross production minus any write-offs, discounts, etc. These are the real dollars that are owed and you have the ability to collect.

Tracking collections allows you to see how effective you are in managing your **Accounts Receivables**. This category tracks the money that is owed to the practice, which is commonly broken down by current and intervals of over 30-days, 60-days, and 90-days. The goal is to see the majority of money that is owed to the practice in the "current" category. When balances creep into the "30-day," and especially the "60-day" and "90-day" categories, your chances of ever collecting that money dramatically decrease.

Remember, you are only as successful as what you collect!

Since the hygiene department is the engine that keeps your practice moving forward, it is important to track how many patients have been pre-appointed for their next hygiene appointment. The goal of the Practice Growth System is to ensure that every patient will ALWAYS have an appointment in your schedule. It is much easier to take on the task of pre-appointing patients during their appointment when they feel the most value for your services. Once a patient leaves the office, the importance of getting their teeth cleaned drastically changes to a medium or low priority.

Keeping track of new patients is also critical to the growth of your practice because without a consistent influx of new patients, your practice will begin to slowly die. It also is important to monitor attrition or patients that have left the practice. It's simply part of the dental business that patients will leave your practice for a variety of reasons. However, the only way to really know that you are providing the best customer service possible is to know the exact reason a patient chose to leave your office. This information will allow you the opportunity to continue to improve the dental experience you are offering to your patients and dramatically reduce the percentage of patients transferring to another office. I know this can be an uncomfortable task. Many of us want to ignore this statistic because it's painful to hear that a patient was unhappy. However, the "leader" inside of you must step up, put your ego aside, and learn from these situations.

Lastly, we want to monitor the number of **Charts Audited**. As diligent as your team might be in keeping patients in the Practice Growth System, some patients inevitably will fall out of the system, but they still need to be accounted for. Most practices attempt this task once every few years or not at all, and this is far too important to ignore. The "charts audited" category determines the growth opportunities available to you and should be addressed regularly. It's critical to have an accurate count of all active patients, meaning a count of all patients who have visited your practice in the past year or year and a half. Why have a room full of patient charts when the majority of those charts are inactive? If we know how many patients are in our practice, then we can accurately determine the correct number of team members to support those patients and the amount of production we can expect from this group. Without knowing this number, we are simply left to guessing.

There is another report that will allow you to take an even more detailed look into your practice. I recommend running the Practice Analysis Report from your dental management software at the end of each month. This report will give you a detailed breakdown of your gross production for the month, along with the individual production categories, so you can see exactly what procedures are making up your total production number. This is important because often we might think, for example, that we are doing tons of root canals when in reality it only averages one per month. This can be extremely important information, especially if you are considering investing $50,000 in an endo-only microscope!

Practice Success Monitors are an essential tool to help simplify the management of your practice. They are easy to understand and will keep you on top of the financial aspects of your practice.

DR. MICHAEL DOLBY

LEADERSHIP

Practice Made Perfect
Blueprint for a Successful Dental Business

DR. MICHAEL DOLBY

LEADING YOUR TEAM TO GREATNESS

Leaders are not born; they are made.
And they are made just like anything else—through hard work.
And that is the price we'll have to pay to achieve any goal.
—Vince Lombardi

5 ESSENTIAL TRAITS OF AN EFFECTIVE LEADER

Confidence

A Clear Vision

Excellent Listener

Elevates Potential

Walks Their Talk

At some point during your career, usually while struggling to motivate your team to support the vision of your practice, you will ask yourself this question: *"Do I have what it takes to lead my team?"*

So I ask you this: *"Are leaders born or are they created?"*

It's an interesting question because I think the majority of us want to believe that leaders are born. We want to accept this belief mainly to compensate for our own lack of effective leadership. We tell ourselves that we are unfortunately not born to be leaders. It is true that some people display leadership skills earlier than others; however, I believe that everyone can be an effective leader in his or her own way. So, are leaders born or are they created? The answer is both. I believe everyone is born with the tools to *learn* how to become a great leader.

Have you ever witnessed that some people can walk into a room and own it? Their presence takes over, they seem bigger than life, and they appear to be true leaders—without saying a word. What is it about these people who command such a presence with what appears to be little effort?

The answer is—confidence. Please don't confuse this with cockiness or arrogance. Confidence is the first of the Five Essential Traits to becoming an effective leader.

CONFIDENCE

Confidence is the state of absolute certainty. This doesn't mean that you know the answers to everything. It means knowing who you are, where you are going, and what you are about. That is ultimate confidence.

I mentioned the importance of "certainty" when presenting treatment plans. Presenting with no doubts or hesitations portrays confidence. Confidence begins with your body language or nonverbal communication. The way you hold yourself will show the world your level of confidence. Here's an example: Imagine someone who stands tall and proud. Then compare that to someone who is slumped over with a blank stare on their face. When you feel good about yourself, you walk a little taller and with a jump in your step. When you are sad or in a depressed state, you look down, move slowly, and speak quietly.

An effective leader displays confidence to the team with both words and body language. No one wants to hitch their wagon to someone who is unsure of what they are doing, where they are going, or what type of practice they are trying to create. Indecisiveness will kill your efforts of becoming an effective leader of your team. Consistently showing confidence is the first step toward leading your team to greatness.

A CLEAR VISION

A clear vision reveals to your team the culture you want for your practice. It represents your brand, the quality of care, the goals of the practice, and what is expected of each person on the team. Without this clarity, your practice would have a tendency to become whatever the latest dental trend is. Choose a vision that reflects who you are, not what you think you should be. Start by deciding what you like and what you don't like. If you can't stand it when a patient comes in with jaw pain, then advertising TMJ therapy services and promoting night guards is probably not going to work out so good for you. The same can be said for cosmetic dentistry. I believe most dentists feel pressure from our industry leaders to offer cosmetic treatments. However, if you believe that peoples' smiles are perfect just the way they are, then promoting veneers would not be something you would want to spend your time or marketing dollars on. You won't feel comfortable presenting this type of treatment anyway, and your patients, along with your team, will detect this insincerity.

Decide what you truly enjoy doing; then put together a framework for the vision of your practice. Once your vision is created, you can build on all of your systems, including your team, around the vision you have created and begin to develop a practice that perfectly fits you and your beliefs and values.

EXCELLENT LISTENER

When we think about communicating between people, who do you think has the "active" role in the conversation? Would you say it's the "speaking" role or the "listening" role?

If you decided that listening is the active role, you would be correct. However, most people just assume the speaking role is the so-called "active" role because that is the one actually talking. In our busy world today, many people, when they are in a conversation and supposedly listening, are really selfishly thinking only about their next statement, with little regard about what the speaker is saying. You can imagine just how much a person with this habit would miss in a conversation.

Listening means paying attention, not only to the story, but how it is told, the use of language and tone, and how the other person uses their body. In other words, it means being aware of both verbal and non-verbal messages. Richard Branson, the CEO of the Virgin Empire, frequently quotes listening as one of the main factors behind his success.

The first step in becoming a great listener is making the conscious decision to become one. A great listener takes in all the information they hear and is well aware they don't have all the answers. By listening intently, you may hear an idea that you have never considered before. When you find yourself in the listening role, make sure your mind doesn't drift. Remind yourself to stay focused on what the speaker is saying. Once you have decided to make this a priority in your life, then you will see immediate improvement in your listening and retention skills.

Dentists who lack good listening skills and believe they have all the answers, unfortunately, end up leading their team with a "my way or no way" attitude. They soon find themselves with a group of employees who are mentally and emotionally checked out. The practice becomes just a job for the team members, so they just punch the clock and do the minimum amount of work to get by. The uneducated dentist will immediately blame the team, thinking they are all lazy, but the problem is actually right under the dentist's own nose!

In order to become a great leader for your practice, you can start by becoming a great listener. Actively listening to your team and to the ideas they have of how to make improvements in the practice is a great start to transforming a group of employees into a true TEAM.

ELEVATES POTENTIAL

Have you ever watched a football team with players who individually were average athletes at best yet seem to consistently win? I mean, on paper these guys would be considered too small, too slow, and not strong enough. However, with the right coach and working as a team, they become absolutely unstoppable, where no one can beat them!

How does this happen? How does a group of average players defeat a group of superstars? The answer is: a great leader. Great leaders will elevate the potential of their team to actually perform above their natural ability. When team members are told they are great consistently and reinforced by training and practice, their performance can be simply amazing. They are able to reach levels of success they would never be able to achieve on their own. I have witnessed teams that even when they were down, just knew with absolute certainty they were going to rise above the temporary setback and achieve victory because everyone on the team shared this same belief.

You can accomplish this phenomenon in your dental practice. With confidence, a clear vision, and great listening skills, you can elevate the potential of your team to one that will reach unstoppable heights. It's up to you to create a culture where your whole team believes that together they are the best.

WALK YOUR TALK

I have found that people who tend to brag about how successful they are often have some of the least successful businesses. Great leaders don't have to tell everyone how great they are because their actions speak for themselves.

The final trait to leading your team to greatness is that you must Walk Your Talk. You must live by, not just the words you say, but also your actions. I've seen dentists preach punctuality while consistently arriving late to exams and team meetings. If you are the last one to arrive at the office and the first one to leave, you forget to return phone calls to patients, and you reschedule team meetings because of conflicts in your personal schedule, then don't be surprised when your team members start showing the same behaviors.

It's impossible to be a great leader if you create rules and guidelines for your team that you have no intention of following yourself. With this type of "Do as I say and not as I do" attitude, your team will naturally mimic your behavior while ignoring the vision of the practice.

Your personal work ethic will set the tone for the culture that is created in your practice. Your team cannot do this for you. It must come from you—the leader of the practice!

ANNUAL PLANNING MEETINGS

You don't have to see the whole staircase; just take the first step.
—**Martin Luther King**

Why do we throw anniversary parties or celebrate birthdays? We do this to recognize special occasions that honor a great year or a significant milestone in our lives. So why don't we consistently do this with our business?

Annual planning meetings are a great way to celebrate the successes you have accomplished throughout the year. It can be a great opportunity to reflect on the practice as a whole and to thank your team for all their efforts. These types of formal meetings are really essential to your overall growth and are certainly not reserved for just the big multi-doctor offices, as some doctors believe.

The primary reason annual planning meetings are not conducted with predictability is because many doctors view them as unnecessary and unproductive. *Why pay the team for a feel-good meeting if it's not going to make the practice more profitable?* This type of thinking could not be further from the truth. Taking the time to plan and review the year ahead and, more importantly, to celebrate the success you and your team have experienced is absolutely the best thing you can do to continue the growth of your practice.

Most annual planning meetings fail because they are not well organized or thought-out. Without structure and specific goals in mind, the meetings will likely turn into a brief and general review session of how the practice has been performing. Unproductive tangents can take over and waste everyone's time, with no chance for growth opportunities for your practice or your team.

A well planned, strategic annual planning meeting is very important for your business and provides the opportunity to recognize the successes and challenges you have seen throughout the year. Celebrating the hard work of individual team members and planning for the year ahead make invaluable tools. These meetings give your team the opportunity to renew the vision and mission statements of the practice, set new goals for the upcoming year, and develop or enhance each department's business systems.

Consistent strategic meetings elevate your practice to a higher level of performance. This is your chance to end poor performances and welcome a brighter future.

I have outlined how to plan your next productive and successful annual team meeting:

MAKE THIS A MANDATORY MEETING

To get the most out of annual planning meetings, you must make it mandatory for ALL team members. You can schedule this meeting during the week when you are not caring for patients or even over a weekend. However, your entire team must be present and ready to contribute.

It is appropriate to compensate your team for this meeting. This can be either at their normal hourly wage or a predetermined non-clinical wage, such as when you are traveling as a team to continuing education meetings. When you compensate your team, they feel appreciated and willing to participate and make the meeting as productive as possible. If you do not compensate your team, they most likely will just go through the motions and count the minutes until the meeting ends, resulting in a waste of time for everyone.

Don't try and schedule annual planning meetings after a half-day of caring for patients. Your team will most likely be tired and have trouble focusing on the important topics. The more time and effort you put in to making this a special event, when people are at their best, the more your team will respond with excitement and enthusiasm.

Determine Your Location

If possible, schedule your meeting at a location other than your office. This will emphasize the importance of the meeting to your team. It could be a meeting room at a hotel, a nearby resort, or a restaurant with a large banquet room that you could reserve for the day. You want to choose a location with little distractions so that you can be as productive as possible. Be creative and make this a memorable event that your team will look forward to each year.

Be Prepared

The most productive annual planning meetings are guided by a detailed agenda that will allow your team to move quickly through everything you want to accomplish. It's important to include team-building games to keep the meeting active and break up the heavy business talk. The best meetings will mix business with FUN, so set your lab coat aside and have a good time!

Learning new business systems to make your practice as efficient as possible can take time, and it's important to review these systems periodically throughout the year and especially during your annual planning sessions. I have seen teams that over time incorporate improvised versions of the original system, ultimately leading to failure. Team members have told me, "Oh, yeah, we used to do it like that," but they aren't sure why they ever stopped. The great John Wooden said, *"It's all about fundamentals,"* so plan to consistently review and master the systems in your practice in order to keep moving forward towards your goals.

Below are just a few business system examples you can review at your next annual planning meeting:

Soft Tissue Management Program
Clinical Efficiency
Effective Case Presentations
Team Job Descriptions
Financial Arrangement Options
Proactive Case Presentations
Introduce New Technology
Marketing Plan
Outstanding Customer Service
Bulletproof Re-Care Program
Scheduling for Maximum Profitability
Office Design and/ or Decor

Encourage Brainstorming & Contribution

Brainstorming is a great way to create new practice-building ideas as a team. When your team is involved in creating better and more profitable ways to conduct your business, they will tend to honor those goals.

Begin by choosing three or four areas that your practice needs to improve, and list them on a sheet of paper with three blank lines after each for team members to give their ideas. It's important to let your team know there is no such thing as a bad idea. So give them permission to open up and be creative.

Make your team part of the annual planning process by assigning certain portions of the meeting's agenda for a particular team member to prepare and present. For example, this might include a more efficient way to answer the phone or a better way to care for emergency patients. It can be an invaluable learning experience for each team member to explain the day-to-day duties of their individual department to the rest of the team. It's important for everyone on your team to know the specific duties of every department in order to clearly understand the challenges each department faces. This also identifies pitfalls and opens up opportunities to offer assistance by fellow team members.

I love the story about a dental assistant who believed that her job and the detailed organization she put into it was the absolute toughest of all the jobs in their office.

After a few months, a change of team members resulted in her moving to the position of front office manager. This job was nothing like she had ever experienced, with phones ringing and patients constantly needing her attention. She soon decided that this indeed was the toughest job of all.

After a few years, she missed the clinical aspect of dentistry and went back to school to become a hygienist. In this position, she found herself hunched over all day trying to convince her patients that bleeding gums are not normal, and then went home at night exhausted both physically and emotionally. Now she was absolutely certain this job was definitely the toughest in the office.

Finally, she decided that what she really wanted to do was become a dentist. So she enrolled in dental school and after graduation started her own practice. She treated patients, managed a three-person team, struggled to keep the practice profitable, went home exhausted, and ultimately decided that THIS was by far the toughest job in the office.

I love this story because it's normal to feel that your job is the toughest of all! In fact, all jobs in the dental office require hard work if you operate at a level that demands exceptional customer service and give attention to every detail while producing the highest quality care possible. Every department relies on the other, so it's beneficial that everyone on the team understands the unique challenges that each one of these departments faces.

With this insight, your team will become more efficient and productive, working together to make each department better, instead of thinking they have the toughest job of all.

Have Fun!

Annual planning meetings should be a day of celebration, brainstorming, building strong bonds among team members, and having FUN! Incorporate games and activities throughout the day. Your team will be more engaged in the serious topics and leave at the end of the day motivated to capitalize on their goals first thing Monday morning.

TEAM PERFORMANCE EVALUATIONS

There is no passion to be found playing small—in settling for a life
that is less than the one you are capable of living.
—Nelson Mandela

Team performance evaluations are an essential part of leading your team to greatness. This is your chance to step up and show that you are the leader of your practice and, more importantly, that your team can count on you. These evaluations play a significant role in the professional development, performance recognition, and reaffirming the vision and goals of the practice for every team member.

Successful performance evaluations should involve interactive and open communication, and should be an enlightening experience for everyone. These reviews in no way should be intimidating or degrading. The goal is to help team members understand their roles in the practice and what is expected from them based on their job descriptions. They should be recognized for the things they are doing well and informed of areas where they need improvement.

Prescheduling Team Performance Evaluations

Always preschedule the date and time of performance reviews. If you inform your team members the night before, it will only create tension and resentment, resulting in a stressful and counterproductive review process.

Decide how many times per year you want to conduct performance reviews. While some practices hold one comprehensive evaluation per year, other practices choose to conduct informal or "mini" reviews two to threes times a year, along with a formal year-end review. This strategy can be very beneficial, especially with a newly formed team that requires more communication. It will also provide you the opportunity to get to know your team members a little better. This individual attention is a way to show team members they are valued and taken seriously.

Mini reviews do not include salary negotiations. You want to address working conditions, future opportunities, problems, and solutions for improving the practice, etc. These evaluations can be quick, taking only 15 to 20 minutes. They are simply an informal "checking in" review. Take notes on a mini-evaluation form, so you can refer back to this information during the yearly formal evaluations.

Effective Team Member Evaluations

The setting for performance reviews should be a place where team members feel comfortable. Sometimes the doctor's private office can make team members feel as if they are being sent to the principal's office. If you feel this might be the case, choose a neutral place, such as the reception or break room, and you will find your meeting will be less tense and more productive.

Your review questions should not be institutional, as this will just come across as impersonal. It's important to be sincere and understanding when it comes to your team member's perspective of the challenges they face with their position. These evaluations should be filled with praise and provide suggestions for improvement. It doesn't matter if this is your "star" team player; there is always room for improvement.

Make sure that all of the information gathered during this evaluation is documented, so there is never a misunderstanding. Document your employees' reactions and attitudes during the reviews. Are they present, engaged, and willing to do the work necessary to excel? If an employee's answers and body language are telling you he or she is checked out, this might be a good time to decide if this is the right person for your team. I have seen dentists keep team members onboard, even when they knew it was the wrong match, because it was just too uncomfortable to let that person go. The longer you keep a team member who doesn't support the vision of the practice, the longer it will take you to reach your goals.

It's important to keep the process moving forward, so you are able to cover everything efficiently in one hour or less. Remember to focus on the big picture of giving each person the support and tools to help them meet the goals of the practice.

Self-Performance Evaluation Form

I am a BIG fan of team members evaluating themselves before a review. All too often during the review process team members find themselves just sitting and listening quietly as the doctor does all the talking, and they never seem to get an opportunity to present their own opinion. Your main goal during the evaluation process is to clearly understand how your team members view their contribution to the practice. By providing them the opportunity to share that information, you will get far more out of your performance evaluation.

Encourage your team members to be open and honest when writing a self-evaluation. Their comments should be turned in one week before the scheduled evaluation, so you have adequate time to review their specific issues. This allows you time to address your concerns and the concerns of your team member. When people feel they are being heard, they feel respected. When they feel respected, team members will develop an "ownership mentality" to the practice.

Team Member Compensation Evaluation

Dedicate a significant portion of your scheduled evaluation time towards compensation, especially detailing the team member's total compensation package. Often team members only see their hourly wage and forget about bonuses, profit-sharing, or health insurance, etc. All of these extra benefits add significant expenses to the practice and must be shared with your team members, so they have a clear picture of exactly what they are receiving. This will give them the opportunity to completely understand the true value of their compensation package.

The evaluation process will be more effective when the following are included:

Team members are encouraged to review their job descriptions beforehand.

This gives them an opportunity to really evaluate what they do for the practice and make any changes to their job description or refresh what has previously been outlined for their position. It's important for every team member and the doctor to know exactly who is responsible for what, so accountability can be established.

Team members complete the self-evaluation forms before their reviews.

The self-evaluation form is an opportunity for team members to share their ideas and challenges, and to provide an honest evaluation of their performances. *(You may find that they will actually be harder on themselves than you.)*

Goals outlined.

The team member's goals for the year should be clearly outlined in the evaluation areas for improvement, acknowledging good performance and establishing new expectations.

Don't do all of the talking.

Remember, listening is the power position. Ask your questions and give your team members an opportunity to respond, sharing their feelings and telling you what challenges they are facing.

Provide opportunity for disagreement.

If you come to a point of disagreement that cannot be resolved, provide the opportunity for your team member to have their opinion heard and documented, and set a later time and date to review this. This will give both of you time to properly evaluate the concern and possibly come to an understanding.

Put your team members at ease.

To have a productive review, your team members must be able to contribute to the process. If they are nervous or scared, they won't be able to communicate their concerns.

Give praise.

Everyone needs to be recognized for their contributions to the practice. Make sure adequate time is spent focusing on what they are doing right.

The evaluation of team members is an ongoing process. Take notes throughout the year and reflect back on the "mini reviews," so that nothing is missed. Your goal is to clearly assess the way your team member is performing in relation to their job description and requirements.

Remember to preschedule team performance evaluations and prepare properly to ensure that you will have a productive meeting. An honest evaluation includes job performance and achievements. You may have opinions regarding the employee's home life and personal choices, but don't let this influence your evaluation of how they actually contribute in your practice.

Finally, it's important to keep the evaluation process relaxed and comfortable. No one should feel intimidated or abused. These reviews should be beneficial to everyone and build a solid working relationship with team members. The evaluation process is a valuable tool to improve the productivity and environment of your practice. Great leaders commit to mastering this process.

Team Member Performance Evaluation Form

Name: _____ Position: _____ Date: _____

1.   Clearly defined role in the practice:

   N/A   Unsatisfactory   Needs Improvement   Good   Exceptional

2.   Committed to Mission and Vision statements of practice:

   N/A   Unsatisfactory   Needs Improvement   Good   Exceptional

3.   Consistently takes action to achieve practice goals:

   N/A   Unsatisfactory   Needs Improvement   Good   Exceptional

4.   Starts and ends on time each day:

   N/A   Unsatisfactory   Needs Improvement   Good   Exceptional

5.   Contributes to morning and monthly meetings:

   N/A   Unsatisfactory   Needs Improvement   Good   Exceptional

6.   Challenges self to improve every day:

   N/A   Unsatisfactory   Needs Improvement   Good   Exceptional

7.   Understands the Practice Growth System:

   N/A   Unsatisfactory   Needs Improvement   Good   Exceptional

8.   Customer Service:

   N/A   Unsatisfactory   Needs Improvement   Good   Exceptional

9.   What is your greatest strength and weakness?

10.   What can we do as a team to improve our practice in the next three months?

11.   What challenges are keeping you from meeting your goals?

12.

Individual Performance Evaluation Form

Name: _____ Position: _____ Date: _____

1. Describe your defined role in the practice:

2. State the Mission and Vision Statements of the practice:

3. Consistently takes action to achieve practice goals:

   N/A   Unsatisfactory   Needs Improvement   Good   Exceptional

4. Starts and ends on time each day:

   N/A   Unsatisfactory   Needs Improvement   Good   Exceptional

5. Contributes to morning and monthly meetings:

   N/A   Unsatisfactory   Needs Improvement   Good   Exceptional

6. Challenges self to improve everyday:

   N/A   Unsatisfactory   Needs Improvement   Good   Exceptional

7. Understands the Practice Growth System:

   N/A   Unsatisfactory   Needs Improvement   Good   Exceptional

8. What challenges are keeping you from meeting your goals?

9. What is your greatest strength and weakness?

10. What can you do in the next three months to improve the practice?

11.

Team Member Compensation Review

Team Member Name: _____

For Calendar Year Ending _____

The following is a complete breakdown of your total compensation package.

Your contribution to this team is extremely valuable, and we find it very important that you know what is included in your total compensation package.

Hourly Wages/Salary .... $_____

Bouses... $_____

Health Insurance .... $_____

Medical Reimbursement/Cafeteria Plan........................... $_____

Health Savings Account (HSA) Contributions........................... $_____

Retirement Plan Contributions .... $_____

Continuing Education .... $_____

Other:_____ .... $_____

Total Compensation and Benefits .... $_____

Total Hours Worked.. _____

Total Compensation and Benefits Per Hour .... $_____

TEAM HANDBOOK

To know what people really think, pay regard to what they do,
rather than what they say.
—**Rene Descartes**

An important communication tool between the owner of the practice and team members is a well-structured team handbook. This will set forth the expectations you have for the team and describe in detail what they can expect from you as the owner, along with addressing the legal obligations you have as an employer and outlining your team members' individual rights.

Team handbooks are necessary to address the significant policies, practices, and procedures in your office. Everyone on your team must be required to familiarize themselves with the contents of the handbook when they are hired. The handbook is designed to summarize practices followed most frequently in the normal course of operations, but it is not intended to be inclusive of commonsense policies. The purpose is to give team members a clear understanding of what is expected of them and what they can expect of the practice. These policies and procedures are intended to promote a safe, equitable, friendly, and enjoyable working environment that complies with federal and state laws.

Nondisclosure agreements (NDAs) are not required by law, but when employees are asked to sign NDAs, conflict of interest, or non-solicitation agreements, it can help to protect the unique way you run your practice, as well as the private information that is discussed among your team.

Your employee handbook must state that you are in compliance with the equal employment opportunity laws that prohibit discrimination and harassment, along with being in compliance with the Americans with Disabilities Act.

A team handbook should be simple and direct, providing answers for your team regarding every aspect of their employment. Listed below are few of the highlights you should consider:

Salary and Payroll Policies

Clearly outline pay periods and probationary timelines for paid benefits. Explain that your company will make the required deductions for federal and state taxes, and voluntary deductions for profit-sharing programs, if applicable. In addition, you should outline your legal obligations regarding overtime pay, continuing education compensation, salary increases, time-keeping procedures, breaks, and bonuses. The more detail you can have, the less headaches you will experience as the years click on.

Work Schedules

Describe in detail your company's policies regarding work hours, schedules, attendance, punctuality, and the reporting of absences. Leave no doubt about the time your morning huddles begin and the flexibility of when your day ends. Don't assume that your team members will respond to everyday challenges in the same way as you would. Clearly outline your expectations and guidelines, so there is no room for misinterpretation.

Standards of Conduct

Describe in detail your expectations of how you want your team members to conduct themselves, including dress code and ethics. Remind your team members they are representatives of the practice while they are in the practice and even after hours, outside of the office. They should conduct themselves with the same integrity and professionalism that is expected when they are caring for patients.

General Employment Information

Your team member handbook should include a summary of your business employment policies covering employment eligibility, background checks, job descriptions, team member referrals, records, probationary periods, dress code, and termination procedures, etc.

Safety and Security

It's very important to define your policy for creating a safe and secure workplace. Include compliance with the Occupational Safety and Health Administration's laws that require team members to report all accidents, injuries, potential safety hazards, and health- and safety-related issues. Describe your policy on locking up the office at the end of the day and a detailed buddy system, if applicable. Safety policies should include your company's policy regarding locking file cabinets, HIPPA laws, and commuting to work in bad weather.

Computers and Technology

Outline policies for appropriate computer, phone, and software use. In our world of digital communication, it's important to address this topic in detail, so you don't have team members constantly checking their phones throughout the day. To account for HIPPA regulations, describe steps team members should take to secure electronic information, especially personal identifiable information you collect from your patients.

Team Member Benefits

Detail all benefits offered by the practice and the eligibility requirements for those benefits to take effect. Outline your plans for optional benefits, such as health insurance, retirement plans, holidays, bonus plans, continuing education pay, and wellness programs.

Leave Policies

Company leave policies should be carefully documented, especially those you are required by law to provide. Family medical leave, sick leave, jury duty, military leave, and time off for court cases and voting should all be documented to comply with state and local laws.

Team member handbooks might feel like a pain in the butt, but they are essential for every practice. There are many companies that will create this for you, but beware of using one that is so generic that it doesn't pertain to your practice.

TEAM BONUS SYSTEM

By working together, pooling our resources, and building on our strengths,
we can accomplish great things.
—**Ronald Reagan**

A dentist friend of mine told me the story of how he wanted to take his practice to the next level. To do this, he was going to create a bonus system that would motivate his team to work harder and increase production and collections.

He designed a separate plan to reward the front office for increased collections and another plan for the clinical team to increase production. The team seemed to love the idea of growing the practice and had high hopes of making a little extra cash. However, after just three months, neither the production nor collection goals were being achieved, and the practice was in a steep decline. To make matters worse, the team was at odds with each other. The front office was pointing fingers at the clinical team, and the clinical team was blaming the front office for not reaching their goal.

Instead of bringing his team closer together and growing the practice, he now had a massive breakdown in relationships and trust. The bonus system was quickly discontinued, and it took months, along with some changes in personnel, to get the team back on track.

The majority of dentists want to reward their teams for a job well done. They set out with the best intentions in place and create a bonus system. However, often these bonus systems are tied to individual performances and do not consider the team element that is critical for any growth in the practice. When constructed this way, these types of bonus systems will do more to destroy the team than bring it together.

In order for a bonus system to be successful, it must contain three key elements:

(1) Easy to Understand. Team members must know exactly what it will take to make a bonus and approximately how much that bonus will be worth.

(2) Reward Equally. It is absolutely critical to reward your entire team equally when the goal is reached. The plan that was described above failed because it rewarded individuals and disregarded the team effort behind reaching those goals. The fact is, it takes the entire team to complete a crown, root canal, root planning, etc. In order for a patient to receive a new crown, they must first be in rapport with the doctor and the team. The crown is diagnosed by the doctor and usually supported in the hygiene department. Financial arrangements are made with the front office, the patient schedules their appointment and the dentist completes the crown with the help of an assistant. This is certainly a TEAM effort, so for a bonus system to be successful, it must reward the entire team as a whole because everyone on the team plays an essential role in achieving the bonus goal.

(3) Celebrate Together. When a bonus is reached, the team must be able to celebrate together. When bonus payouts are rewarded equally, it's easy to celebrate together. However, if the hygienist's bonus check is twice as much as the assistant's, the assistant is going to feel slighted, and morale will suffer.

Bonus systems should be based on some sort of a rolling average of your production and collections. If your bonus system is based solely on month-to-month calculations, the practice could be in jeopardy of paying bonuses for productive months while struggling financially during the down months. It is crucial for the long-term success of the practice that a bonus is paid out to team members only when the practice is profitable. With that said, the system that I have found to work the best is calculated each month and based on a three-month rolling average of net collections, total team compensation, and team overhead. The key to this bonus system is determining the percentage of your total team compensation as it relates to your office overhead.

For example, most peak-performing practices set their total team compensation to not exceed 20 to 24 percent of their total office overhead. When that number is established, as production increases a bonus is paid for any collections exceeding the 20 to 24 percent number. So if the total team compensation for the three-month rolling average come out to be 18 percent of total net collections, then the team would see a bonus pool of 2 to 6 percent, depending on what percentage of total team compensation was chosen. This bonus pool would then be divided equally among team members, based on hours or days worked.

To determine the "overhead" number of your bonus calculation, simply decide on what percentage you want for the team's total compensation as it relates to overhead. For example, if you want to cap the team's total compensation at 20 percent, then you would divide 100 by 20, and your "overhead number" would be 5. That will be the number used in your bonus calculations.

In the example below, we are considering the months of June, July, and August. We have listed the net collections *(what you put in the bank)* along with total team compensation for those months. Be sure to subtract any previous bonus money paid during those months from the total team compensation, so that you are not penalizing your team for making a bonus the month before. Calculate the average for the net collections and total team compensation. Those numbers, along with your pre-determined overhead percentage number, will be used to determine if bonus dollars have been achieved.

This form is easy to understand and can be used by anyone in the office. In fact, you should encourage all of your team members to get involved with these calculations. The more your team can get excited about increasing production and increasing collections, the more bonus money they will likely see while making the practice grow.

Team Bonus System

August 2013

Month	Net Collections	Total Team Compensation
June	$73,394	$15,565
July	$82,435	$14,320
Aug	$88,303	$14,020
TOTAL	$244,132	$43,905

Total Team Overhead = 20% or 5.0 *(100 / 20 = 5.0)*

Total Team Compensation x Overhead Number
equals Bonus TOTAL (BT)

$43,905 x 5.0 = $219,525 (BT)

Total Net Collections - Bonus Total / 3 (months)
= $ Average for 1 month, Divide by Overhead Number = $ Bonus Pool
/ Number of days worked = $ Bonus per Day

$244,132 - $219,525 = $24,607 / 3 = $8,202 / 5 = $1,640 / (16 days) = $102
Net Collections   Bonus Total   month's   overhead   **BONUS**

Every team member would receive a bonus of $102 per day, multiplied by the number of days they worked that month. You may notice the bonus check totals may be different totals because it would not be fair if a part-time employee, working eight days per month, makes the same as someone who is fulltime, working 16 days per month. The daily bonus is the same, just the amount of days worked is different. Instead of using days worked, you can also choose to break down this total to hours worked for the month, essentially coming up with roughly the same number.

AVOIDING UNHAPPY PATIENTS AND POTENTIAL LAWSUITS

*As you grow older, you'll find the only things you regret
are the things you didn't do.*
—Zachary Scott

What if a loyal patient, one whom you have given your very best efforts, decides to file a complaint with the dental board and a lawsuit because their dentures don't look natural?

Naturally, you would be disappointed and possibly think that you're not a good dentist or even worthy to practice dentistry. However, we know that nothing could be further from the truth. The fact is, great dentists get sued just like anyone else, and over the course of a 30- or 40-year career, I can almost guarantee that someone, for some reason, will challenge your treatment choices and possibly file suit. Lawsuits are a scary thing, but if you are prepared, it doesn't have to be a nightmare.

There is a reason they call it a "dental *practice*." It is not a perfect science, and we shouldn't expect perfection. A new crown on patient "A" is not even close to the same procedure as a new crown for patient "B." Each person we care for brings a completely different set of circumstances, and we can even go so far as to say that each tooth we treat will present its own set of challenges.

Complications with treatment happen to all of us. How we handle these temporary setbacks determines whether our experience is positive or negative. Fortunately, if you incorporate a few simple tools into your practice, they will dramatically reduce the risk of an unhappy patient or an unfortunate lawsuit.

TLC CALLS

"TLC" post-op calls are one of the most powerful ways to let your patients know that you care about them. The fact is, that when you are in rapport with your patients, they are going to be less likely to file a lawsuit if something happens to go wrong. In other words, if they like you, they probably won't sue you. So our goal is to deliver such outstanding customer service that every patient is considered a friend.

The system is very simple to execute and is probably the biggest practice-builder you could ever do to accelerate the growth of your business. Every patient who receives anesthetic during treatment must receive a personal phone call later that evening from the doctor or the hygienist, depending on who performed the treatment. You are simply checking in to find out how they are feeling and to ask if they have any questions or concerns until you see them again. It's just that simple!

A personal TLC call will set you apart from all other health care providers. Your patients will know that your concern for them extends far beyond their office visits. I have been following this system for the past 20 years, and I'm still amazed when patients tell me they have NEVER had a doctor call to ask how they were doing after treatment. It is a powerful gesture that, unfortunately, is not used consistently in most practices.

Some practices will try and delegate the task to an office manager or assistant. This may be better than not making a call at all; however, it doesn't have the same effect as when the call comes from the doctor. These calls only take 10 or 15 minutes at the end of your day and create more practice-building rapport than you could ever achieve with an unlimited marketing budget.

Dentists often ask me if they should make these calls for minor treatments, such as a buccal pit. My answer is always a resounding Yes! If your patient was numb when they left your office, then they need to hear from you. From your patient's perspective, anything they have done in your office is never "minor treatment," so this call is just as important from a patient's perspective as if you extracted a tooth. The fact is these are the easiest calls to make because you already know that your patient will be feeling great.

TLC calls will also decrease the number of emergency calls you receive after hours. When you reach out to your patients in this fashion, more than likely you will have answered any of their questions, and they will wait until the next business day to address if they need to be seen.

It is easy to set your practice ahead of the rest by incorporating a TLC call system into your practice, but remember—CONSISTENCY is the key to its success.

FINANCIAL ARRANGEMENTS

Most dentists have had a patient who calls, after hours, about a cavity diagnosed three years before that now needs a root canal. You leave your family, rush to your office to get them out of pain, and they show you an overwhelming amount of appreciation. Then they get your bill ...

It is amazing to witness how much value is lost once a patient is out of pain and their focus switches to the $2,000 bill for a root canal, buildup, and crown. Your patient might even go as far as to look for things that aren't *"just right"* with the treatment and delay or refuse payment.

Most patients have no clue how much dentistry costs, and if they have dental insurance, they think everything is completely covered. So when there is no prior discussion about their out-of-pocket expense, you leave the door wide open for your patient to feel jaded about the treatment you recommended for them.

No one likes surprises when dealing with money, so it's crucial to always tell your patient what they are expected to pay at the time of treatment, along with what you estimate their insurance benefit will cover. Even with emergency treatment, provide your patient with at least an inflated estimate, so they have some idea of the costs they are about to incur. Pain has a way of superseding the cost of emergency treatment; however, an estimate of fees will go a long way to help preserve the relationship and avoid surprises once they are able to think more clearly.

I always suggest presenting treatment plans as the worst-case scenario *(under promise/ over deliver.)* That doesn't mean everything ends with an extraction and implant, but if their tooth has deep decay, then you would be wise to prepare your patient for the possibility of a root canal. This will at least inform them there is a strong possibility of more extensive treatment if they want to save their tooth. If the treatment happens to be less than anticipated, there is nothing better than telling your patient the treatment cost was actually less than expected. This is a very important strategy to use because when treatment plans change, as they may, in the patient's mind they will think you (1) didn't do a good job diagnosing from the start or (2) you screwed something up! Again, under promising and over delivering will set you free from upset and legal action.

The team member who presents treatment plans MUST explain the value of the treatment to patients. If the treatment plan is presented in a monotone or unemotional manner, your patients will likewise show little excitement. Imagine if you buy a new car and the sales person throws you the keys and says, *"I hope you like your new car."* You just paid a significant amount of money, and they deliver it to you as if you possibly made a bad decision. Compare that with my experience buying a Prada purse for my wife. The salesperson set the purse on a cashmere cushion, as if it were the Hope Diamond, and then wrapped it in a Prada box that looked like it cost as much as the purse itself. It made us feel as if we made a great decision and bought something of high quality that we valued.

What if the dental treatment you recommend is presented with this kind of enthusiasm and presentation? Your patients would follow your lead and also feel a great deal of value for the treatment you are recommending. Remember, people won't buy anything they don't VALUE, regardless of whether they have the money or not. If enough value is created, your patients will find a way to afford anything you propose.

When financial arrangements are addressed before treatment and you have prepared your patients for the best- and worse-case scenarios, no matter what path the treatment takes, you will have preserved your relationship and professional integrity. If you are not willing to address finances upfront, you might as well prepare to write off the treatment you just performed—along with your patient!

CONSENT FORMS

Consent forms are a great way to make your patient take ownership for their decision to proceed with the treatment you have recommended for them. Lawyers recommend that all dentists use consent forms because if you are sued, the attorney for the plaintiff will certainly ask, *"Did you properly inform your patient of the their treatment choices?"* and *"Where is the signed consent form?"*

Patients have the right to accept or deny proposed treatment, and a consent form provides them that opportunity. These forms don't need to be complicated, but they must include a few key items in order for the patient to be considered "informed."

The Principles of An Informed Consent

Informed – The patient has enough information to make an educated decision about the treatment being proposed and why it is recommended.

Alternatives – It gives any other choices the patient may have to complete the proposed treatment.

Complications – It tells any negative results that may occur as a result of the proposed treatment along with not following through with the proposed treatment.

Voluntary – The patient has made this decision on his or her own.

Ability – The patient is in the right presence of mind and has the mental capacity to make an educated and informed decision.

All states require that patients be provided with an informed consent before dental treatment is started. Informed consents evolved from the crime of "battery," which is basically the unauthorized touching of another person. A landmark case from New York in 1914 laid the foundation for informed consent, stating: "Every human being of adult years and sound mind has a right to determine what shall be done with his own body; a surgeon who performs an operation without his patient's consent commits an assault, for which he is liable in damages." (*Schoendorff vs. Society of NY Hospital; 211 NY 215; 1914*)

The purpose of a consent form is to confirm that the patient knows exactly what treatment they are agreeing to have you perform and they have enough information to make an educated choice, along with understanding the alternative treatment options. Without a consent form, patients may claim they didn't completely understand the treatment proposed or the alternative treatment options, especially if complications arise.

A patient with pain may elect quickly to remove their tooth rather than have a root canal, buildup, and crown. Some people choose what seems like an immediate fix without a complete understanding of the possible effects from their decision. For example, this might create a change in their occlusion, drifting teeth, or increased sensitivity. Dentists have the responsibility to inform patients of any possible complications along with viable solutions.

I recommend using a detailed consent form for all oral surgery, implants, root canal therapy, and periodontal surgical procedures. In my private practice we use a general consent form that is signed by the patient during their new patient introduction to the office, which informs them that we will be performing all procedures to the current standard of dental care determined by the State Board of Dentistry. This will cover you with your more basic procedures such as fillings, cleanings, etc.

REFUSAL OF TREATMENT

Not every patient is going to agree with every recommended treatment plan you present. Often the refusal is a byproduct of the dentist's not being in rapport with that patient. However, when a patient decides not to complete their treatment, dentists are required to share more information regarding the risks associated with this refusal. Patients must have a clear understanding of the risks and consequences of their decision. Sometimes dentists must explain the same outcome in different ways, so they are confident the patient is making an educated decision.

What should you do when all the explanations of the proposed treatment have been exhausted? A dentist has two choices: Continue to treat your patient with the limitations they have placed on you, or dismiss the patient from your practice because it would be impossible for you to provide quality dental care within those limitations.

Both choices unfortunately, have positive and negative ramifications. For example, if you choose to continue treatment without proper x-rays, then you are liable if something goes wrong, even in the future. *(The dentist in this case would be taking all the risk because patients cannot legally consent to a dentist's negligent act)*, and if you choose to dismiss the patient, you risk harm to your reputation.

Always make the professional choice to continue with the patient's best interest in mind, operating at or above the standard of care. No one benefits if you compromise your treatment procedures, no matter what the reason. I recommend looking at each case individually. Ask yourself one question: "Does the patient's refusal of treatment directly affect the level of care that I provide?" If the answer is "yes" *(and most likely it will be)*, then you should remove yourself from their care and assist them in finding another dentist.

Some dentists will chase money and take on a case when they don't have the proper experience, and naturally those decisions will increase the likelihood of a bad outcome. I can assure you that no case is worth compromising your patient's safety or risking a lawsuit. If it doesn't feel right, acknowledge that feeling and do not move forward. Never take on a case if you cannot make a significant improvement or if you are limited in your choice of diagnostic instruments or tools.

If you cannot build value for your treatment plan and a patient still insists on refusing, then your only choice is to ask them to sign a refusal of treatment form. You may be surprised by their response. It's not uncommon for a patient to change their mind and now accept your recommendations because they finally understand how serious you are about their health and your unwillingness to compromise your standard of care.

However, if a patient refuses to sign the refusal form, you can sign the form yourself and have your assistant *(or whoever was in the treatment conference with you)* also sign as a witness, where the patient was supposed to sign. You can write, *"Patient refuses to sign form."*

It is important to complete this step because, in many situations, this may be the conclusion of your professional relationship. If any legal action takes place, you can be assured that you have taken the appropriate steps to protect yourself.

EXAMPLE

Informed Consent for Dental Treatment

The dental treatment that is necessary to treat my existing oral condition(s) _____
_____ has been explained to me, and I have had the
opportunity to have my questions answered.

Procedures, alternatives, and complications have been discussed, including the
consequences of no treatment.

I understand that dentistry is not an exact science and success cannot be guaranteed.
I also understand the results of my examination, the proposed treatment(s), possible
complications, and the anticipated results.

I authorize Dr. _____ and/or such associates and assistants as may
be necessary to perform the following procedures: _____
_____
_____
_____

This includes the administration of any anesthetic *(including Lidocaine, Septocaine, etc)*,
analgesia *(laughing gas)*, or other medications or pharmaceutical agents *(drugs)* that
may be necessary. I realize and agree that changes in my treatment *(such as a larger
filling)* may be necessary.

I voluntarily assume any or all possible risks that may be associated with any part
of these procedures. I understand it is my responsibility to diligently follow the
postoperative instructions given to me in regard to my treatment.

Patient Signature: _____ Date: _____

Signature of Guardian if Under 18 y/o:_____ Date: _____

Doctor's Signature: _____ Date: _____

<u>EXAMPLE</u>

Refusal of Treatment

Patient's Name _____ Date of Birth _____

I am being provided a treatment refusal form, so I may fully understand the treatment recommended and the consequences of my refusal. I have been provided with enough information, in a way that I can understand, to make a well-informed decision regarding my proposed treatment. I understand and have been given the opportunity to ask any questions I wish regarding this recommended treatment.

Nature of the Recommended Treatment

It has been recommended that I have the following treatment: _____
_____

This recommendation is based on visual examination(s), on any x-rays, models, photos, and other diagnostic tests taken, and on my doctor's knowledge of my medical and dental history. The treatment is necessary because of: _____
_____

The intended benefit of this treatment is: _____
_____

Alternative Treatments

The treatment recommended for me was chosen because it is believed to best treat my particular case. I understand that alternative ways to treat my dental condition include:
_____

Risks of the Recommended Treatment

I understand that no dental treatment is completely risk-free and that my dentist would take reasonable steps to limit any complications of my treatment. I understand that some after-treatment effects and complications may occur. These include:_____

Risks of Not Having the Recommended Treatment

I understand that complications to my teeth, mouth, and/or general health may occur if I do NOT proceed with the recommended treatment. These complications include:_____

DR. MICHAEL DOLBY

Acknowledgment

I, _____, have received information about the proposed treatment. I have discussed my treatment with Dr. _____ and have been given an opportunity to ask questions and have them answered. I understand the nature of the recommended treatment, alternate treatment options, and the risks of the recommended treatment and my refusal of care, and I do NOT wish to proceed with the recommended treatment.

Signed: _____ Date: _____
Patient or Guardian

Signed: _____ Date: _____
Treating Dentist

Signed: _____ Date: _____
Witness

CASE SELECTION

Most dentists have experienced patients who have arrived at their office carrying pictures of a movie star or model and are hoping that you will make their teeth look just like the celebrity's teeth. They are extremely motivated and ready to open their checkbook; however, what they are really asking is for you to make them look EXACTLY like this movie star, in terms of body, hair, face, etc.—you get the picture. I realize this can be a very tempting situation to a dentist who is just starting to grow their practice while sitting alone in their office because of the third no-show of the day. However, we must remember the Three Golden Rules of treatment selection: (1) You don't have to treat everyone; (2) Only accept cases in which you have proficiency; (3) If you can't make a significant difference, then don't start the case.

Carefully selecting the treatment and patients you choose to care for will dramatically reduce your chance of an unfortunate outcome or lawsuit. The only way to know if you can meet or exceed your patient's request is to ask very detailed questions. You must completely understand their motivation to look a certain way, and it is your job to establish reasonable expectations and outcomes, before any treatment begins. Once you have committed to the case, the results will be judged by whatever vision was in your patient's head, so be sure that you are VERY clear about that vision.

I have declined several cosmetic and restorative cases because the expectations of the patients were far beyond what I believed I could achieve. When the best-case scenario is not enough to make the patient happy, your best move is to walk away. Tell the patient that due to the complexity of the case, you don't feel that you would be the most qualified to take care of them. This way you don't burn bridges or make them feel as if they are being unreasonable—even if they are—and, more importantly, you can preserve the relationship and your name.

DOCUMENTATION

The documentation of your chart notes for each patient is really only important when a transferring dentist asks for your records or you are called to present this documentation in a lawsuit. Wow, those are pretty good reasons to make sure you have a system of accomplishing great chart notes. You can imagine that either of these situations would be a very humbling experience if your chart notes were incomplete or vague. We have all heard the saying, *"If it isn't written, it didn't happen."* Accurate and complete chart documentation is truly the single most important item you have in the event of a malpractice claim or patient complaint. Getting lazy in this area of your practice may end up costing much more than you ever dreamed!

I met a dentist once, who early in his career made a habit of entering his chart notes at the end of each day, instead of after each patient. However, when his practice became busier and his system of chart entries remained the same, he soon found himself documenting all chart entries at the end of each week. Now I think we can all agree that even with the best memory, a dentist cannot accurately describe the treatment provided to 30 or 40 patients the previous week.

I'm often asked if someone other than the dentist can take on the task of entering the chart notes. My answer is an absolute, yes! If a dental assistant and hygienist are trained properly, they are more than capable of entering accurate and complete chart notes. Provide them with a format to follow, and you will probably find their entries are done with much more accuracy and detail than you did previously.

Whoever is responsible for documentation, it is crucial to document the exact treatment performed, along with the conversations you have with patients pertaining to their treatment. Your chart notes should accurately describe the treatment procedure you performed, so that anyone who reads these notes could recreate that procedure. By creating a system of entering chart notes as part the scheduled procedure time, you will ensure that all chart entries are detailed and accurate. When you master clinical efficiency, you will find there are plenty of opportunities to accomplish this task in the allotted appointment time. When the treatment is complete and before you walk the patient to the front desk to "close the loop," all chart notes, lab slips, etc. should be completed.

There are three items that all chart notes must have in order to be considered complete. They must be:

(1) legible,

(2) credible, and
(3) logically sequenced

Probably the most common problem with chart notes is that they are simply not legible. If nobody can read what you have documented, then it's as if it never happened. You cannot go into a deposition and claim, *"But this is what I really meant …"* That simply won't fly. A normal person must be able to read what you have written. Thank goodness the majority of documentation is taking place on the computer today, so we can eliminate in most cases the fact that many of us have sloppy writing skills, which brings us to our next challenge: credible.

I think we can all agree that chart notes must be deemed credible. What I'm making reference to is the special abbreviations that are common with most dental chart notes. I'm not talking about LOL or OMG, I'm talking about staying with abbreviations that are common in the practice of dentistry. Using abbreviations, such as MOD or OHI, would be considered completely acceptable, but when abbreviations, such as PNC, start showing up (for "patient noncompliant"), it probably won't work. Keep your abbreviated words to a minimum and stay with the most common in the industry.

Chart notes must follow the same sequence as you performed in the treatment. Seems reasonable, right? However, I have read chart entries that were all over the place, describing the impression first, before the crown preparation, and then completely forgetting to mention the temporary. Obviously this is an example of poor documentation. Simply start from the beginning of your treatment sequence and describe what you did until you were done. Note any vital signs you might have taken and note whether or not you described the procedure to the patient prior to starting. Tell if you used topical. Also note the type and amount of anesthetic and what injection technique you used. Describe the actual dental treatment you completed, noting any buildups, near pulp exposures, the amount of decay found, shad of the restorative material and/ or crown, any compromises, all the way down to the temporary material chosen, and even the temporary cement. Be sure to note your post-operative instructions and any prescriptions you may have written. The more detail you can provide here, the better. However, keep this in perspective—you don't need to write a book for every procedure you do. You simply need to recreate what you accomplished, so another person can have a clear understanding.

There will certainly be a time when you need to make a change in your chart notes or you may have forgotten to add an important detail. This is not a problem, as long as you go about making this entry the correct way. First and foremost, never attempt to erase, white out, or alter in any way previously written chart notes. If you need to "add" something to the chart notes, you can simply create a new dated entry, including your initials, and address your concerns. If the previous entry was just completely wrong, you can draw a single line through the entry with your initials and then document the correction.

The SOAP sequence of chart note documentation seems to work, even with today's modern practices. This is a simple system to keep your chart notes consistent. This outline should precede your progress notes or the actual treatment you performed.

S   O   A   P

Subjective
Describe the purpose of your patient's visit, which includes areas of discomfort, pain, duration, general symptoms, etc.

Objective
Your assessment of your patient's situation, describing things that can be measured, seen, felt, touched, etc.

Assessment
This refers to the diagnosis from the dentist regarding the patient's condition.

Plan
This refers to the treatment plan that has been decided by the dentist and the patient.

Your completed progress notes would follow your SOAP evaluation, with a detailed description of exactly what occurred during the treatment, regarding materials, methods, and procedures.

PRACTICE TRANSITIONS

*It takes 20 years to build a reputation and five minutes to ruin it.
If you think about that, you'll do things differently.*
—**Warren Buffett**

Imagine you have just spent the past 30 years caring for your patients, watching many of them grow up, go to college, or get married. Now it's time to say goodbye. Transitioning your practice to someone else can be more of an emotional challenge than a business one.

Dentists, who retire, not only struggle with the reality they won't be caring for their patients anymore, but an even bigger struggle is the emotional loss of their identity. If you are no longer a doctor treating patients, then who are you? This emotional challenge forces many dentists to continue practicing well past the time when they should retire. They no longer have the energy to be productive, and the value of their practice tends to decline rapidly.

Practice transitions can be the best or worst experience of your career, and it greatly depends on who you have by your side guiding you through this emotional business journey. A strategic plan must be implemented before a potential buyer is determined. The most important element of a successful transition is creating a win-win situation for everyone involved: the selling doctor, the new dentist, your patients, and your team members.

I think we can all understand the emotional struggle that retiring doctors face, but we must remember the team also faces these same emotional challenges. Think about it, they have been by the dentist's side for most, if not all, of the dentist's career, and they are very likely to experience the typical phases of grief—denial, anger, bargaining, depression, and acceptance—so it's important to recognize and expect these feelings. The more communication you have with your team during the transition process, the smoother the experience will be for everyone.

I remember a dentist who once, without much consultation or advice, decided to sell his practice. He was burned out and looking for immediate change. His practice was one that most dentists dream of owning with annual production averaging $1.3 to $1.45 million while only working Monday through Thursday. To make things even better, this was an insurance-independent office with accounts receivables averaging a mere $2,000 to $4,000 a year. This practice was simply amazing in all aspects of the business along with its reputation in the community, and, not surprisingly, it sold for the full asking price within two weeks of the listing.

The purchase and sale agreement allowed the selling doctor to work two days per week for the first year to assist with the transition of the new doctor into the practice. Unfortunately, like most plans that don't have a coach or a mediator to keep both parties on track, egos soon got in the way, and not long after the sale, it was clear the new doctor had a deep desire to be ruler of his own domain. The transition process quickly began to collapse, and the agreement for the selling doctor to work two days per week promptly ended.

When the selling doctor departed, so did most of the existing patient base. The mass exodus was so large, the new doctor had to hire a fulltime person just to handle the number of patient transfer requests. Nearly half of the original patient base left the practice, and many of the remaining patients were on the fence about whether to stay or go. This was certainly not the outcome that anyone envisioned or wanted.

The importance of a well-thought-out transition plan cannot be overstated enough, and it begins with qualifying the buyer. When you finally decide to list your practice for sale, just because a buyer arrives with cash in hand, it doesn't mean they are the right fit for your particular practice. With a proper evaluation, the buyer in the above story would have been identified as a bad fit, and both doctors could have avoided this unfortunate transition experience.

I have purposely used the word *"transition"* to describe this process of changing doctors/ owners. Many practice brokers will use the word *"transaction"* because to them this is nothing more than a quick sale and a commission. The word *"transition"* acknowledges how delicate this process can be and the individual attention that is required, so that buyer and seller both receive maximum value.

Six Essential Principles of an Effective Transition

Discovery

Preparation

Valuation

Qualifying

Transitioning

Support

DISCOVERY
The Game Plan

Discovery is the process of understanding the culture of the practice. This is a key element in determining the right type of buyer for a successful transition to occur. Discover how the practice is viewed in the community. Discover what specialty services are offered and what makes the practice stand out. The goal is to have a clear understanding of the doctor, the practice, the patients, and the team. The more that is known about the culture of the practice, the easier it will be to find a dentist who will continue with that culture, preserving the patient base and, most importantly, continuing the growth of the practice.

Determining the business cycle of the practice will not only help establish a value for the practice, but it will identify the correct type of candidate that will best fit the practice's needs. Is the practice in a growth phase, or is it stagnant? Has production been declining over the past few years with little effort to correct the downturn? What opportunities are there for immediate and long-term growth? What types of services are offered, and, more importantly, what services are being referred out of the practice? Answers to these types of questions will help to determine the health of the practice and identify new opportunities the new doctor can capitalize on.

Finally, it can be extremely beneficial to know the real reason why a doctor is selling their practice. You must understand exactly what the seller is hoping to accomplish from the sale and, more importantly, their plans after the sale. I cannot overemphasize the importance of having an exit plan. With the example I shared, that doctor was clearly not ready to sell his practice, and with proper discovery, he would have realized the motivation for selling was not congruent with his long-term plans.

The more you can discover about the practice and all of the components that make up the business, the easier it will be to find the correct candidate to fill the role of the retiring dentist.

PREPARATION
Creating the Maximum Value

Many doctors make the assumption their practice is worth much more than it actually is, relying on nothing more than previous years' production numbers. The fact is, your dental practice is worth only what the market will pay at the time of sale. Now many factors will have an influence on the price, such as location, years in business, number of active patients, production, collections, and so on, all of which can dramatically affect the final purchase price of the practice. However, in order to maximize the value of your practice, the first thing you need to do is get it ready to sell. This may include minor cosmetic improvements, such as painting, changing the carpet, upgrading to hardwood floors, or a thorough floor-to-ceiling cleanup. Introducing proven business systems so the practice is operating at peak performance will all help to improve the bottom-line, making your practice more attractive to a potential buyer.

Unfortunately, most dentists make the decision to sell their greatest investment with little to no preparation or "cleanup," and then they are shocked to discover the value of their practice is not what they expected. Before the practice financials are evaluated and production numbers are reviewed, your office must look its best to realize its maximum value. The easiest place to start and the one thing you have complete control over is making sure the office space is clean.

Doctors are always amazed when I say this, but I consistently walk into dental offices and find tons of clutter: stacks of old magazines in the reception room, furniture that looks like it was purchased at the secondhand store, fake plants with just enough dust, so you know they are fake, and landscape pictures from the 50s decorating the walls! The treatment rooms have everything you could possibly use for just about any procedure proudly displayed on the counter, creating nothing more than clutter, which screams disorganization.

Buyers want to purchase successful practices they can grow, not rebuild from the ground up. Just as if you were selling your home, you want to make the buyer's decision to purchase your practice an easy one, so their first impression is critically important. So make certain the general feeling of the office is up-to-date and ready to present to a potential buyer. *"You only get one chance to make a great first impression."*

Next, you want to address the business side of the practice—the team, production, collections, re-care, insurance, and accounts receivable, etc.—all must be evaluated and improved if possible, for a quick sale and maximum value. Buyers are attracted to practices with business operations that are organized with effective business systems in place and a history of steady growth. Dentists that are heading towards retirement often make the unconscious mistake of devaluing their practice through steadily declining production, increased treatment referrals, and more time spent out of the office, all which can dramatically affect the end value of the practice.

It's not unusual for the preparation phase of a successful transition to take six months to three years to properly implement. Doctors who take this time to prepare their practice for sale can easily add an extra $100,000 or more to the sale price, along with a rejuvenated team that will be ready to take their new doctor and practice to the next level.

VALUATION
Benefiting Both Doctors

There are many strategies for determining the value of a dental practice. The primary goal is to make certain there is maximum value for the buyer and seller—the first step in creating a win-win transition.

Regardless of what the valuation process is called, they tend to fall into one of three categories.

Asset-Based Valuation: With this strategy the value is based entirely on the hard assets of the practice: delivery units, chairs, office equipment, etc. The value can be based on the original cost, appraised value, or replacement value of all the tangible assets of the practice. The obvious shortcoming of this strategy is that there is no consideration of the practice earnings, cash flow, or goodwill. I realize it can be hard to establish a value for goodwill, but the financial impact of what the practice is generating in income must be considered when determining a value for the practice.

Market-Comparison Valuation: This strategy considers what other similar practices have sold for in the area, much like "comps" in selling a house. Several factors are considered when determining valuation, such as cash flow, annual net production and annual net profits, location, active patients in the practice, equipment, etc. It's important to note that no two practices are alike, so the unique features must be identified in order to determine a value for those features.

Income-Based Valuation: This strategy of valuation is based upon the projected future cash flow of the practice. The cash flow is then capitalized, discounted, or multiplied based upon one of the following methods: (1) the present value of future earnings, (2) a capitalization of excess earnings, and a multiple of discretionary earnings valuation. This income-based valuation approach is popular because it recognizes the practice's potential for continued success. The valuation is determined based on the realities of income, expenses, and the anticipated personal income for the buyer.

Other items to consider in the valuation process:

* Past three years income statements and tax returns
* Past three years production and collection reports
* Past three years accounts-receivable reports
* Past three years balance sheets and profit & loss statements
* Current practice analysis
* The *accurate* number of "active" patients
* List of contractual insurance arrangements (HMO, PPO, etc.)
* Equipment condition and value
* Clinical supplies
* Leasehold improvements and copy of lease agreement
* Non-compete agreements

QUALIFYING
Finding the Best Buyer

Now that you have discovered the culture of the practice, made the necessary cosmetic improvements to the office, enhanced the business operations, and established an appropriate value, it's time to find a qualified buyer.

Selling a dental practice is not the same as selling a car. More than likely, the selling dentist will remain living in that community and on occasion will run into former patients, so the level of patient care and customer service within the practice must not be compromised in any way. The selling doctor's reputation in their community is going to be very important to them. Therefore, a qualified buyer would be one that presents with the clinical skills and mindset that fit the existing culture of the practice. Can you imagine selling a high-quality cosmetic practice to a dentist who believes every person's smile should be left in its natural state, regardless of what the patient wants? This person would obviously not be the right match. Selling dentists must take as much time as needed to find the "right" person, so he or she can exit with dignity and respect.

All too often, I see doctors try and hide from their team members the fact their practice has been listed for sale. I assume they think the team's knowledge may in some way compromise the sale, when in fact quite the opposite can occur when you involve your team. Let's face it—they are going to know anyway, so just let the cat out of the bag and make them part of the process. The reality is, they are going to be the ones left to work with the new doctor, so allowing them to have an opinion during the process can go a long way in creating a successful transition.

TRANSITIONING
Preparing Your Team

The majority of team members will get the sense when their doctor is about to retire. When that time comes, expect that some of your team members will not react as positively to the change in ownership as you would like. The fact is, most people don't handle change of any kind very well, so it's important to involve your team in the transition process as early as possible. Team members really want to know that their positions in the practice are secure and that the new owner will be a good person to work for. Preparation and planning to lessen the impact and uncertainty of this transition are critical to preserve the good will of the practice.

Just as patients look to assistants, hygienists, and the front office team members for confirmation regarding treatment options, they are also going to look for that same support during the transition of a new doctor. When the team has been included in the process and properly prepared, they will be excited about the new opportunities ahead, and patients will share in their excitement. Team members will need to emphasize the positives of the transition, such as extended office hours, new treatment opportunities, or extended emergency hours, to every patient, so they too can accept and embrace this change.

INFORMING YOUR PATIENTS
Celebrating

When you have found the perfect candidate to take over the reins and they have the support of your team, it will be time to inform your patient base. The goal of an official announcement to patients is to create excitement and celebration, not mourning the departure of the retiring doctor. Let's face—it most patients are going to be mostly interested in how this change affects them, so give them a reason to celebrate. Patients need to be assured that the level of care and, more importantly, the team members of the practice will remain. When the current team is there to provide comfort and reassurance to these patients, they are much more likely to accept the new dentist.

There are several ways to inform patients that a new dentist is taking over a practice. First, announce the transition a minimum of six to eight months before the new doctor arrives. This allows time to complete a full re-care hygiene cycle where patients can be told in person about the transition of the practice. There is nothing better than informing your patients in person, so you can answer any questions or concerns they have, right there and now. There is nothing worse than letting people create their own stories in their minds, creating more uncertainty and likely resulting in their looking for new dental homes.

During this information period, having a mini resume of the new doctor with his or her picture *(on 4 x 6 cards)* is a great way to inform patients a new doctor will be joining the practice. The postcards can be handed out at the reception desk to all active patients during their re-care visit, along with mailing them to unscheduled or inactive patients. Having something in print, especially with a photograph, goes a long way in motivating patients to accept the new dentist, putting a face to the name. It can be hard for patients to comprehend when told in person or by phone, especially when they are apprehensive about the change. A printed postcard allows them to review the information at their convenience when they are possibly in a more relaxed environment.

A newsletter and or a press release for local newspapers or magazines, announcing the transition, can be a very effective method of informing existing patients. Again, the goal is to create energy and excitement about the transition. The more excited you and your team are, the more likely your patients will follow your lead.

Lastly, hold an open house, so existing patients and the community have the opportunity to meet the new doctor in a relaxed atmosphere. The local chamber of commerce or Better Business Bureau can cosponsor these events, and remember to keep a schedule handy because it's not uncommon to get a few new patients at these events.

Change in any practice can produce some level of anxiety and uncertainty. When patients feel this way, they tend to look elsewhere for dental needs. If you create a feeling of celebration about the new doctor, patients tend to lose that anxiety and uncertainty. Before a candidate is ever established, the team must believe in the change and accept the transition plan. Patients trust team members and will look to them for guidance throughout the process.

TYPES OF TRANSITIONS

There are many transition strategies out there, and while some work well, others don't work at all. I like systems that have proven track records, so consider these two types of transition scenarios:

(1) *The Graceful Exit*: This transition strategy involves selling the entire practice to a new dentist while allowing a strategic four- to six-month transition period to occur. The selling doctor is actively assisting the team and patients during this period while making a graceful exit at a predetermined date. This transition preserves the goodwill of the practice because of the personal transfer or recommendation of the selling dentist to the patient base. Once patients feel secure, they are likely to stay in the practice because their uncertainty is gone. This does require a commitment

on the part of the selling doctor; however, when this type of transition can be utilized, it often results in the best outcome for the new doctor and existing team members.

(2) *The Extended Stay:* Sometimes doctors are not quite ready to walk away from clinical dentistry altogether, but they do want to slow down. Many will decide to sell half of the practice to another doctor who essentially becomes a partner. The senior doctor continues to practice as they grow the office into a two-doctor practice. When the senior doctor is ready to retire, he or she can sell the other half to the existing partner or another dentist. This can be a very profitable strategy for selling a practice because the two halves are likely to be worth more than the original whole, due to the increased value created by another dentist growing the practice. However, you must know this strategy has its pitfalls. First off, you are taking on a partner, and partnerships are notorious for clashing egos and team member challenges. Second, this process can take much longer to mature than expected, so patience is critical for this to succeed. Lastly, it can be challenging to find a buyer for half of a practice because the purchasing dentist is essentially being forced to enter into a partnership. However, this strategy is a great solution for large practices that have a patient base or sales price that is too large for one doctor to acquire alone.

SUPPORT
Continued Success

In this phase, the "correct" dentist has been found and the transition process has gone exactly as planned. Excitement is in the air, and it's not uncommon for the practice to excel during this transition period when patients, doctors, and team members are happy and at peace, with nothing but optimism for the future. Unfortunately, as time goes on, when the energy and excitement from the transition have died down, the senior doctor retires, and the practice either plateaus or begins a gradual decline. A support team or coach can be beneficial to help the practice run smoothly after the senior doctor has retired, so practices don't have to experience a downturn in their growth.

A practice management/ transition support coach will work with the doctor and team through the transition period, checking in with the practice periodically and making sure the business systems remain active and in place, all of which is incredibly beneficial for the continued momentum and success of the practice.

As you can see, there are multiple steps and strategic planning in order to achieve a successful practice transition. Without consideration of this process, this may very well end up being the worst experience of your career. However, when dentists combine the practice management support and implement the Five Essential Transition Principles, both the buyer and seller are certain to experience stress-free and profitable transitions.

THE ETHICAL DENTIST
Setting the example for your team

I hate to even bring up the topic of ethics, but I think it's important for all of us to remember why we got into this profession in the first place and how we should consistently care for every patient we have the honor to care for. Every one of us upon graduation took an oath to do no harm, and although I've never met a dentist who would intentionally hurt anyone, I have seen some who have caused harm in unconscious ways.

The ethical dentist is one who is committed to offering only the best treatment options they have available to them. Treatment recommendations that they would offer to their own family members or someone they care deeply about. The ethical dentist never falls into the trap of assuming a patient can't afford the best of care or that they wouldn't be interested. We have an ethical obligation to allow people the right to choose what is best for them—after all, it's their oral health.

Make a commitment to remove the word "patch" from your dental vocabulary. Dental restorations are either functional or need to be replaced. It's just that simple. During my career, I have seen far too much patching of crown margins when the correct treatment was simply to replace the restoration. I think we can all agree this would never be in the best interest for any patient, as they will only get a false sense of security that everything is fine when likely that is not the case.

Always make ethical decisions regarding treatment and your techniques; in other words, don't make things up. If it's not taught in dental school, a postgraduate program, or a continuing education course, then don't do it! I've seen the craziest restorations throughout my career, and once even got into a debate with a dentist who had placed a composite filling in a patient's tooth without completely removing the old silver filling. Essentially, it was half amalgam and half composite. Now I'd never seen a course for this technique before, and I don't think he had either. When you can step back from every case you complete, saying to yourself, "That is exactly what I would have wanted done in my own mouth," then you have performed at the highest level with integrity. You may have heard the old saying, *"Conduct yourself the same, whether or not someone is watching,"* which essentially means: Always hold yourself to the highest standards whether someone is checking your work or not.

Every dentist in our profession is so blessed to have the skills to perform some pretty cool things for people. Practice the way that best fits your skill level and what you enjoy. Only then will you be the happiest and the most successful.

HEALTHY LIFESTYLE

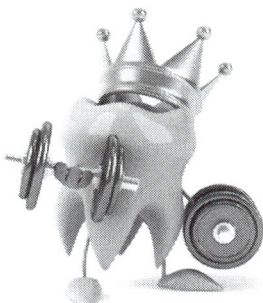

When I was completing my general practice residency program at St. Joseph's Hospital, I had the opportunity to observe a total hip-replacement case. Witnessing this procedure is quite an experience if you ever get the chance. However, as I was watching the orthopedic surgeon position this patient's leg to the left and the rest of his body to the right, essentially splitting him in two, I was amazed to listen to the surgeon complain that he could not see anything. I immediately thought, "Wow, this guy should try performing root canal therapy on a third molar!"

Most people don't realize how demanding dentistry is on a doctor's body. We basically perform microsurgery in an extremely small space, day after day, often putting our bodies in positions that resemble a contortionist. Over time, this takes a physical toll on everything from our joints, back, muscles, etc.

My intention with this chapter is not to inform you about the latest workout fad, or no-carb/ all-carb, no-fat diet. I simply want to open your eyes to the importance of taking care of your body, so that an injury doesn't cut your career short or you end up looking like the Hunchback of Notre Dame when you retire.

YOUR DIET

A diet should not be complicated, but it seems like every week a new diet emerges that is *"the best diet ever created"* and that makes promises that you will lose weight without any effort ... Most of these diets do work for the short term but never seem to last, and most people end up gaining back the weight they lost, essentially creating a yo-yo diet approach.

We all know the importance a diet has in your overall health and vitality. If what you eat is unbalanced in either quality or quantity, naturally this will create an imbalance within your body. I don't think it's any surprise to anyone that today our food contains tons of chemicals disguised as preservatives, flavorings, colorings, emulsifiers, hormones, and antibiotics, as well as residue from pesticides and fertilizers. So it only makes sense to seek out fresh and unprocessed foods to eat whenever possible.

Once you remove all of the fad diets and systems, losing weight is really simple: Burn more calories than you consume. If you follow this rule, you'll NEVER be fat. I absolutely hate it when I hear people say, *"But I'm just big boned, and no matter what I do, I can't lose weight."* Let me ask you a question, "Have you ever seen an overweight person in Ethiopia?" The answer is NO. Unfortunately, many people, who live in the poorest country on the planet, take in fewer calories than they burn. Granted, this is most likely not by choice, but the outcome is the same. If you focus on good nutrition and burn more calories than you consume, then you are likely to experience:

* More Energy
* Improved Sleep
* Less Weight Fluctuations
* Ability to Cope with Stress
* Better Mood
* Better Hormonal Balance
* Less Body Fat
* Improved Sex Drive

Sugar

Most of us know that sugar is not good for our bodies. But did you know that craving sugar is actually built into our DNA? Our ancestors, as they would search for food, learned quickly that sweet foods would not kill them. So, as we have evolved, sweet things like sugar remain in our brains

DR. MICHAEL DOLBY

as pleasurable and safe to eat. It's kind of crazy to think now the thing that we believed would not hurt us is exactly the thing that might be killing us.

Obesity in America is close to reaching epidemic proportions. More than a third (35.7%) of adults and almost 17% of our youth were considered obese in 2009–2010. Not surprising, eighty percent of people with type-2 diabetes, the most common form of the disease, are obese or overweight. The annual medical expenditures attributable to obesity have doubled in less than a decade and may be as high as $147 billion per year, according to a new study by the U.S. Centers for Disease Control and Prevention.

Leading Causes of Death *(CDC report 2013)*

- Heart disease: 611,105

- Cancer: 584,881

- Chronic lower respiratory diseases: 149,205

- Accidents (unintentional injuries): 130,557

- Stroke (cerebrovascular diseases): 128,978

- Alzheimer's disease: 83,767

- Diabetes: 75,578

- Influenza and pneumonia: 56,979

- Nephritis, nephrotic syndrome, and nephrosis: 47,112

- Intentional self-harm (suicide): 41,149

Overeating

Most of us think we overeat because we're hungry. However, it's not that simple. Scientists say the two most important factors that influence how much we eat are visibility and convenience. Have you ever noticed that when a plate of cookies is passed around the table, you grab one without hesitation? This has nothing to do with being hungry—we simply see it and want it!

Here are few simple tricks that could help you lose 15 to 20 pounds per year:

Out of Sight, Out of Mind:
Experts at Cornell University found that when people had a bowl of sweets and chocolates within reach, they ate 125 calories more than when the same bowl was placed just six feet away. Basically, if you put temptation right under your nose, it's harder to resist. If you keep it beyond arm's reach, you'll tend to resist that temptation more often.

Divide and Conquer:
Research shows that we eat 20 to 40 percent more if we serve ourselves or if food is offered in large serving dishes, such as at a buffet. Creating single-portion servings in the kitchen, rather than putting the entire meal on the table and digging in, will also allow you to eat less.

Distracted Eating:
Research published in the *American Economic Review* found that on days when people ate too much, proportionally more of those calories came from foods that were consumed when subjects were doing other things. Several studies have consistently shown that the distraction from television can increase the amount of food you consume. So try to make eating an activity on its own, not something you do at the same time as something else.

Do You Really Know What Hunger Feels Like?
Over the course of a year, if you consume 150 calories more than you need every day, it adds up to an additional 15 pounds you'll put on in that year alone. Before you can begin to control your eating habits, you must learn to recognize the physical cues that signal a real need for nourishment. Before eating any meal, you can use the hunger scale below to help you determine when you reach the "moderately hungry" stage, which is your optimum eating time.

HUNGER SCALE

Starving: An uncomfortable, empty feeling that may be accompanied by light-headedness or the jitters caused by low blood-sugar levels. Your risk of binge eating can double when you get to this level.

DR. MICHAEL DOLBY

Hungry: Your next meal is on your mind. If you don't eat within the hour, you enter dangerous "I'm starving" territory.

Moderately Hungry:

Your stomach may be growling, and you're planning how you'll end that nagging feeling. This is optimal eating time.

Satisfied: You're satiated—neither full nor hungry. You're relaxed and comfortable.

Full: If you're still eating, it's more out of momentum than actual hunger. Your belly feels slightly bloated, and the food does not taste as good as it did in the first few bites.

Stuffed: You feel uncomfortable and might have mild heartburn from stomach acids creeping back up into your esophagus.

STOP AND WAIT!
Understanding Satiety

Your stomach can hold up to about four liters of volume, or approximately 17 cups. However, the feeling of satiety *(the feeling of being FULL)* is not caused by your stomach being full. Instead, feeling full is a result of your brain reacting to chemicals released when you place food and/ or drink in your stomach.

Your brain takes about 20 minutes to register these chemicals. After your meal, the levels continue to rise over 10 to 30 minutes. They stay elevated for three to five hours following the meal, keeping you satiated or feeling full. As the chemical levels fall, the feeling of hunger returns.

The problem with most overweight people is they eat too fast and never give their bodies a chance for the chemical response in the brain to tell them they're full. If you don't feel full directly following a proportioned, controlled meal, then wait. As the level of chemicals increase in your brain, your body will feel full, and your hunger will dissipate.

COUNTING CALORIES

Sometimes meticulously counting calories can feel like the only way to lose weight. However, your body is equipped to know when you have had enough food. By changing your eating habits, listening to your body, and using restraint, you can control your diet by eating the right foods and acknowledging when you are full.

According to the University of Iowa, sedentary women need about 1,600 calories per day, and sedentary men need about 2,200. Your physician can recommend personalized numbers based on your age, health, and activity level.

Divide the amount of calories you need daily by the number of meals you consume. This is the amount of calories you need to sustain your body at each meal. For example, if you eat five meals a day and need 1,600 calories, each meal should be around 320 calories. Either plan your meals ahead of time or count the calories as you go to prevent eating too much. This amount should be enough to keep you full until your next meal, and you can be assured you are not taking in more than your body can burn off; therefore, you will lose weight.

LISTEN TO YOUR BODY

Pay attention to how your stomach feels when you are hungry and then how it feels after drinking a glass of water. The empty sensation should fade slightly within a couple minutes of simply drinking a glass of water. Many times the feeling of being hungry is mistaken for dehydration. Our bodies are about 60 percent water, and that water must be replaced consistently to keep our bodies healthy. Experts recommend that each day we must consume at least 64 ounces or eight glasses of water to remain healthy. Generally, adult males need about 3 liters per day while adult females need about 2.2 liters per day. While some of this water is retrieved from food, we must remind ourselves to hydrate consistently.

Drink a full glass of water 10 minutes before each meal, and your brain will realize you are full within 10 minutes. Have another glass of water with your meal, sipping in between bites to slow your eating. Once you feel full, remove any remaining food from your plate, and engage in another activity, such as reading, conversation, walking, or a hobby.

If you struggle with the urge to continue eating, make yourself a cup of unsweetened tea or coffee, and don't eat again until the emptiness in your stomach returns. Remember the food cravings you experience before your stomach feels empty are mental, not physical, so resist the urge to eat more than your body really needs.

EXERCISE

There are too many exercise routines out there to list, but the important thing to remember is that you must be exercising your body daily. The goal is to have your body moving for 30 minutes a day, five times a week. However, if you are struggling to find 30 straight minutes in your day, you will also experience benefits of exercise even if you divide your workout time into two or three segments of 10 to 15 minutes per day.

Walking, running, and, especially, lifting weights are the best ways to keep your body in shape. Researchers found that muscle tissue burns three times as many calories as fat—and this happens around the clock—yes, even after your workout and when you sleep! That's why you must maintain your strength as you age to keep your body's ongoing fat-burning engine strong.

In the dental profession, the benefits of strong muscles as we manipulate our bodies throughout the day are vast. Here are just a few reasons why:

Help You Lose Weight: Muscle tissue burns as much as 3–15 times more calories per day than fat tissue, even at rest! Nothing heats up your metabolism better than muscle.

Healthy for Your Heart: Your heart can perform better with less oxygen, meaning it doesn't have to pump as hard when you are active and in shape, which means it is less stressed so should last longer.

Protect Your Joints and Your Back: Muscle strength means you put less strain on joints and connective tissue. This is important to dentists, considering the awkward positions we get ourselves in throughout the day. Strong muscles prevent arthritis and career-ending back surgery.

Improve Your Looks: We all want to look good, and lean muscles look better than sagging flab!

Gives You a Mental Boost: You feel energized because of your reenergized metabolic system!

YOGA

This centuries-old, Eastern philosophy of mind, body, and spirit is becoming the new fitness choice for many people. Even prominent athletes are adding yoga to their training regimes to develop balanced, injury-free muscles and spines.

"Americans are usually drawn to yoga as a way to keep fit at first, but the idea behind the physical practice of yoga is to encourage a deeper mind-body awareness," says New York yoga teacher and author Beryl Bender Birch. *"Healing and balancing the physical body helps bring clarity and focus to the mind as well."*

Initially, the sole purpose of practicing yoga was to experience spiritual enlightenment. In Sanskrit (the ancient language of India), yoga translates as "yoke" or "union," describing the integration of mind and body to create a greater connection with one's own pure, essential nature.

If you have never tried yoga or thought that holding your body in different positions was too easy and couldn't possibly be a workout, you might want to take a second look. Yoga is one of the absolute BEST exercises, especially for dentists. The odd positions that dentists and assistants get their bodies into can take an extreme toll on the body. Yoga provides the opportunity to make your body more flexible and strong. Stretching and loosening muscles does a lot to revitalize you after a long week of treating patients.

There are many different styles of yoga, so try a few different types of classes, and you'll quickly discover the right match to suit your needs.

HOW TO GET STARTED?

If you're like most people, you started a diet or workout program with tons of enthusiasm only to witness your motivation disappear. Research shows that 25 percent of weight-loss plans fail within the first two weeks. So how do we stay motivated long enough to see results? The answer is that we must create a habit.

According to Dr. Lawrence Perlmuter, PhD, when you do the same thing for 30 consecutive days, it ingrains and strengthens the brain's neural pathways, so you keep that behavior going on autopilot.

I remember when I was in my second or third year of private practice, working like a madman to grow my practice, and one day I found myself overweight and out of shape. I took my blood pressure, and it was through the roof. If a patient came in with the same reading, I would have sent them to their cardiologist. I was shocked and disappointed in myself. I had been an athlete my entire life, and now my own health was so poor I would actually be turned away for routine dental care. I decided to take action and commit to running five miles per day, five days per week, for one month. At the end of that month, I had a choice: continue with my workouts or quit. As research predicted, I had developed a habit. By the end of that month, I had lost 25 pounds and was healthier and more alert than ever before. The secret is simply starting and committing for a minimum of 30 days!

Start Small: Don't attempt to get in shape in one day. You most likely won't stay consistent, and the habit will not develop. Start small by adding one change per day to your diet or exercise routine. Adding a piece of fruit to your meals while removing the chips, or add taking a walk after lunch—this will go a long way to creating a habit while helping you to reach your goals.

Don't Waste Your Willpower: Avoid temptations. The best way to do this is to stay consistent. Try your best to eat meals at home and not at a restaurant. Strive to work out in the morning before your day begins. I find first thing in the morning is the best time to get a workout in because we all know that once the day starts, it never fails that a meeting or kids' sporting event will take precedent. So give yourself the gift of exercise first, and work second!

Change Your Vocabulary: Be careful with the words you use. Your subconscious only knows your thoughts and has the power to make those thoughts come true. If you think about pigging out in your next meal or that your workout will be painful, that is probably what will come true. However, if you use positive words like "I can't wait to work out" or "This meal is getting me closer to my six pack," it has the power to create the mindset that gives you the subconscious ability to make this actually happen.

Write it Down: As we have reviewed in the chapter about *"Power of Focus,"* writing down your intentions makes them more likely to come true. Write down your weekly and monthly goals, such as eating more whole foods or doing 10 pushups in a row—whatever it takes to keep you moving towards your goals.

Find Support: Find a gym buddy to work out with. It's amazing how we will get our butts out of bed in the morning if our friend is waiting for us at the gym, but we can easily justify sleeping in if it's just us!

Be Competitive: Set goals that will keep you moving in the right direction. I see guys in the gym that arrive at the same time every day, do the same exercises with the same minimal intensity, and see the same minimal results. Hold yourself accountable to make steady progression each week, month, and year.

Everyone must start somewhere. So even if you've been sedentary for many years, today is the day you can begin to make healthy changes in your life. If you don't think you'll make it for 30 minutes, set a reachable goal for 15 or 20 minutes of exercise. You can work up toward your overall goal of 30 minutes by increasing your time, as you get stronger. Don't let all-or-nothing thinking rob you of doing as much as you can every day to make your body as healthy, strong, and fit as it can be!

ERGONOMICS

There is no doubt that dentistry can be extremely hard on your body. As we all know, getting perfect margins doesn't happen on its own, and often we find ourselves in crazy body positions in order to achieve this type of high-quality work. Patients really don't care how hard they make it for us, they only care that the quality of dental work is topnotch, so we end up literally sacrificing our bodies.

When you consider treating patients over a career of 30 to 40 years, giving some attention to the position of your body is an investment that will pay you back your entire career. There are some definite things we can do in the office to keep our bodies pain-free.

CHAIRS

I was one of those stubborn doctors that came from the belief a chair is a chair, and I didn't see the value in spending the money on these so called specialty dental chairs. However, when you think about it, you spend most of your life sitting in this chair, fixing teeth, so it only makes sense that your dental chairs fit your body to provide the least amount of stress on your joints. I often see doctors, assistants, and hygienists in chairs that are old and worn out, and not surprisingly the entire team has some sort of back issue. Don't wait for symptoms to develop, invest in great, ergonomically designed dental chairs, and take care of yourself right now, insuring a long and prosperous career.

MAGNIFICATION LOOPS

Early in my career, my vision was so good up close that I didn't feel I needed any type of magnification glasses. I thought, like many of my colleagues my age, that loops were just for *"old guys,"* and I certainly was not one of them. I remember the day I was working on a patient, and I was so focused on the case that I found myself inching closer and closer to my patient's face, until I was a little too close for comfort, if you know what I mean. I quickly backed off and apologized. Later my assistant told me that I always hunched over like that when I was treating patients!

My team finally got so tired of me running into my office and laying on the floor to ease the pain in my back, they demanded that I try magnification loops that would go out of focus if I started to hunch over or get too close. I discovered that, not only did I avoid any close encounters with my patients' faces, but my posture also improved, and I could actually see everything in so much more detail. This piece of equipment is definitely something every dentist needs, regardless of age!

SLEEP

The old saying, *"I'll sleep when I'm dead,"* may indeed get you there faster than you think! According to one study with over 10,000 participants, there was a two-fold increase in death from all cases of participants who slept five hours per night or less compared to those who slept seven to eight hours. This may be correlated to the fact that sleep deprivation increases insulin sensitivity, which increases risk for weight gain, diabetes, and heart disease. Furthermore, even subtle degrees of sleep deprivation over time can be correlated with immune suppression, cognitive decline, and mental-health problems.

There are two simple things we can do that will have an immediate affect on sleep quality and exercise recovery. First, avoid all caffeine after 3 p.m. Caffeine is a stimulant that stays in your system for more than six hours. Even if you aren't feeling jittery or full of energy, caffeine stimulates the sympathetic nervous system that is associated with increased glucose mobilization, increased blood pressure, and increased alertness.

Avoid using laptops, tablets, and smartphones for at least an hour or two *(or three)* before bedtime. I'm sure all of us are guilty of this, but the intense blue light of these gadgets shines directly into the eyes and confuses the brain. This suppresses melatonin production and disrupts the circadian rhythm, which disrupts your sleep.

Avoiding these and other types of stimuli will allow your body to properly rest and recover, improving your energy and alertness during the day.

THE "PRACTICE MADE PERFECT" DENTIST

Enjoying the Greatest Profession in the World!

I would like to offer my sincere congratulations on your finishing this book. I know that you are a person that has a strong desire to excel and achieve greatness in this profession. The business of dentistry can provide so many gifts to those who choose to maximize their potentials and, frankly, work their butts off! Nothing of any substance ever comes easy, and success in this profession is no different. Applying the blueprint for a successful dental practice based around the three principles of *Foundation, Systems, Leadership™* will certainly get you on your way to being massively successful.

I'll never make the claim to have all the answers, but I have been blessed with a strong desire to keep excelling and growing, both professionally and personally. The knowledge you have gained from this book is just one of the stepping-stones to your amazing career. Continue to challenge yourself, and set goals that will hold you accountable and always keep you moving forward. Tony Robbins once told me that massive change happens in your life from a series of small steps. Individually, they may seem insignificant; however, these small movements are shaping you and your future, so keep pressing on and remember to never, never, never give up.

There is no better time to be a dentist. We have at our fingertips some of the greatest technology in the history of dentistry. We can give our patients smiles that anyone would envy, replace missing teeth with ease, make teeth stronger than ever, and create high-quality restorations chairside. Your practice is the result of all the hard work of becoming a dentist, and you deserve the rewards that business can provide. My hope is that I can *"Elevate the business knowledge of EVERY dentist, so they can experience owning a Profitable, Stress-Free Dental Practice."*

Please feel free to reach out with any questions you may have, and I really hope to meet you in person one day or see you at a live event. Until then, enjoy your gift of being a dentist, the greatest profession in the world!

All my best,

Dr. Mike Dolby

To request Dr. Dolby to speak at your next event:

800-213-0252 (o) 208-866-8092 (c)

P.O. Box 6151 Boise, Idaho 83707-6151

drdolby@triumph-dental.com

For more information and to order additional
Practice Made Perfect books please visit:

www.Triumph-Dental.com

SOURCES

Beryl Bender Birch — New York yoga teacher and author.

Documentation — The Business of Dentistry: Patient Records and Records Management Natalie Kaweckyj, LDARF, CDA, CDPMA, COMSA, COA, CRFDA, CPFDA, MADAA, BA; Wendy Frye, CDA, RDA, MADAA; Lynda Hilling, CDA, MADAA; Lisa Lovering, CDA, CDPMA, MADAA; Linette Schmitt, LDA, CDA, MADAA; Wilhemina Leeuw, MS, CDA

Ferrie, J. E., Shipley, M. J., Cappuccio, F. P., Brunner, E., Miller, M. A., Kumari, M., and Marmot, M. G. "A prospective study of change in sleep duration; associations with mortality in the Whitehall II cohort." *Sleep* 30, no. 12 (2007) : 1659–1666.

Figueiro, M. G., Wood, B., Plitnick, B., and Rea, M. S. "The impact of light from computer monitors on melatonin levels in college students." *Neuro Endocrinol Lett* 32, no. 2 (2011) : 158–63. PubMed PMID: 21552190.

Hartley, S. L., Barbot, F., Machou, M., Lejaille, M., Moreau, B., Vaugier, I., Lofaso, F., and Quera-Salva, M.A. "Combined caffeine and bright light reduces dangerous driving in sleep-deprived healthy volunteers: A Pilot Cross-Over Randomised Controlled Trial." *Neurophysiol Clin.* 43, no. 3 (June 2013) : 161–9. doi: 10.1016/j.neucli.2013.04.001.

Listening — http://www.skillsyouneed.com/ips/listening-skills.html#ixzz3XET522Lb

Napoleon Hill — *"Think and Grow Rich"* - 1937

The McGill & Hill Group, LLC. — 8816 Red Oak Blvd., Suite 240, Charlotte, NC 28217. Phone: 704-424-9780 Toll-Free: 877-306-9780 Fax: 704-424-9786 info@mcgillhillgroup.com

Nehlig, A., Daval, J. L., and Debry, G. "Caffeine and the central nervous system: Mechanisms of action, biochemical, metabolic, and psychostimulant effects." *Brain Res Rev.* 17, no. 2 (May–August 1992) : 139–70.

The Richardson Group — Practice Management Consulting: Fortune Practice Management

Tony Robbins — Robbins Research

Greg Stanley — Whitehall Management. 9815 N. 95th Street, Scottsdale, Arizona 85258. Phone: 480-860-5700 (Fax) 480-451-8102

Today's Dental — Howard E. Farran II, D.D.S. 10850 S. 48th St., Phoenix, Arizona 85044. Phone: 480-359-1352

Valuations — Dentistry IQ: Barry F. Levin. Saul Ewing LLP's Business Department

DR. MICHAEL DOLBY

PRACTICE MADE PERFECT

59826992R00131

Made in the USA
Lexington, KY
16 January 2017